LOOE LIFEBOATS

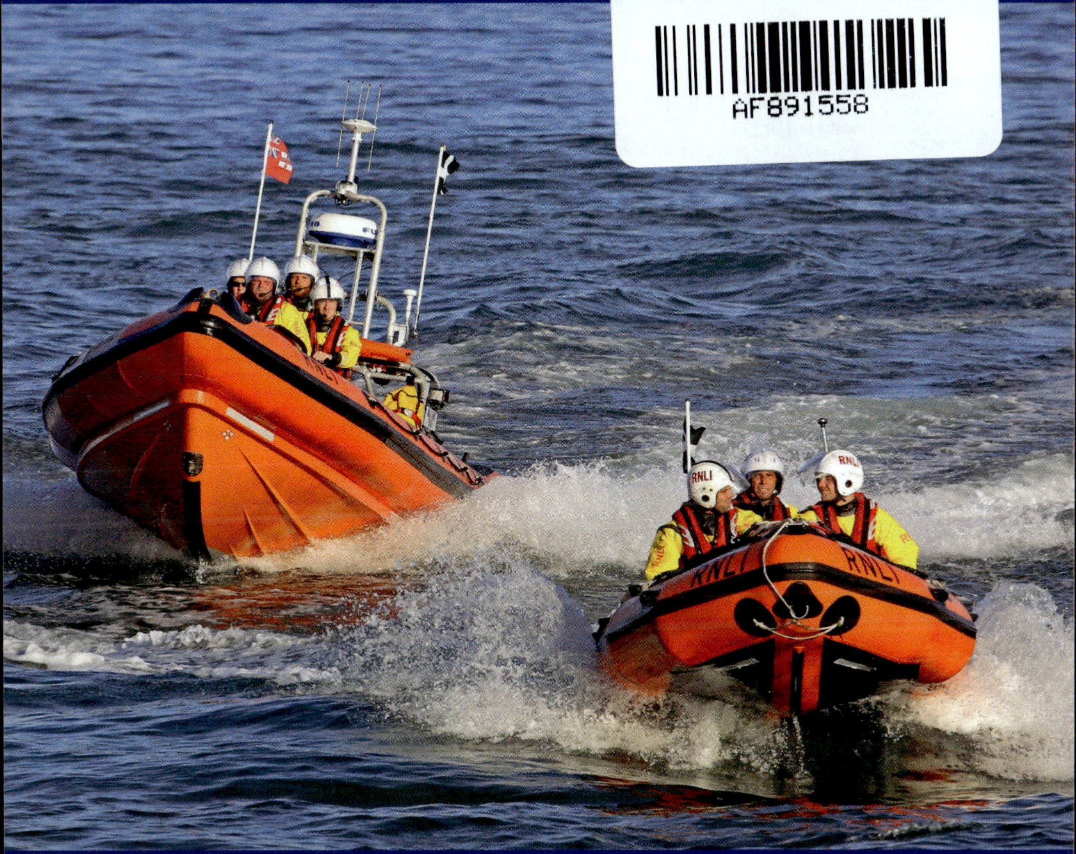

Nicholas Leach

ISBN 9781909540163

• Published by Foxglove Publishing Ltd
• Foxglove House, Shute Hill, Lichfield, Staffs WS13 8DB
• t > 07940 905046, e > njl7@outlook.com
• Layout and design by Nicholas Leach/ Foxglove Publishing

ACKNOWLEDGEMENTS • This book, work on which began before outbreak of the Covid pandemic, could not have been written without the help and support of personnel at Looe lifeboat station, in particular Lifeboat Press Officer Ian Foster, who answered many queries, sent rescue reports, and kindly supplied many excellent photographs for possible inclusion, as well as Lifeboat Operations Manager David Haines, and I am grateful to them both.

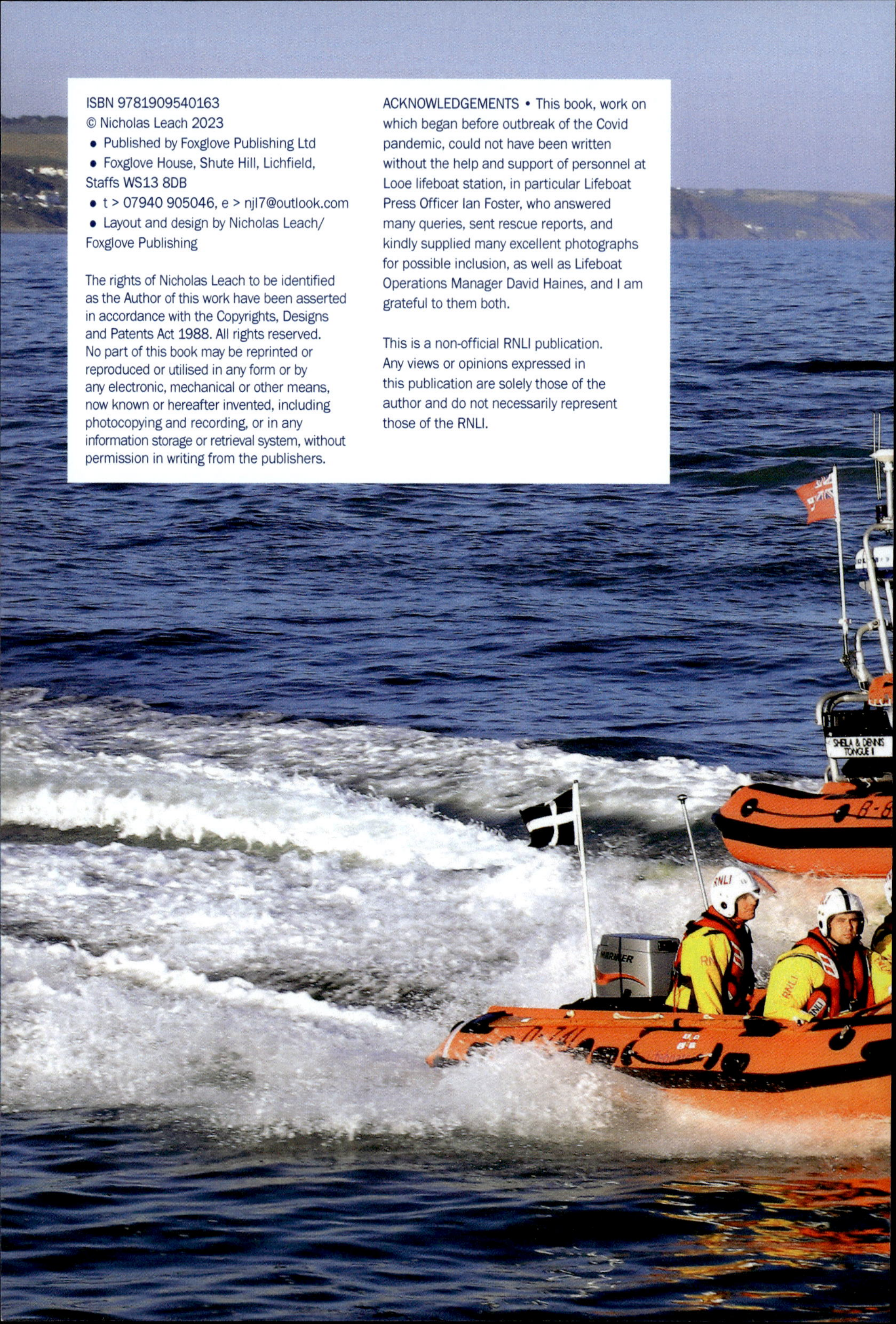

Contents

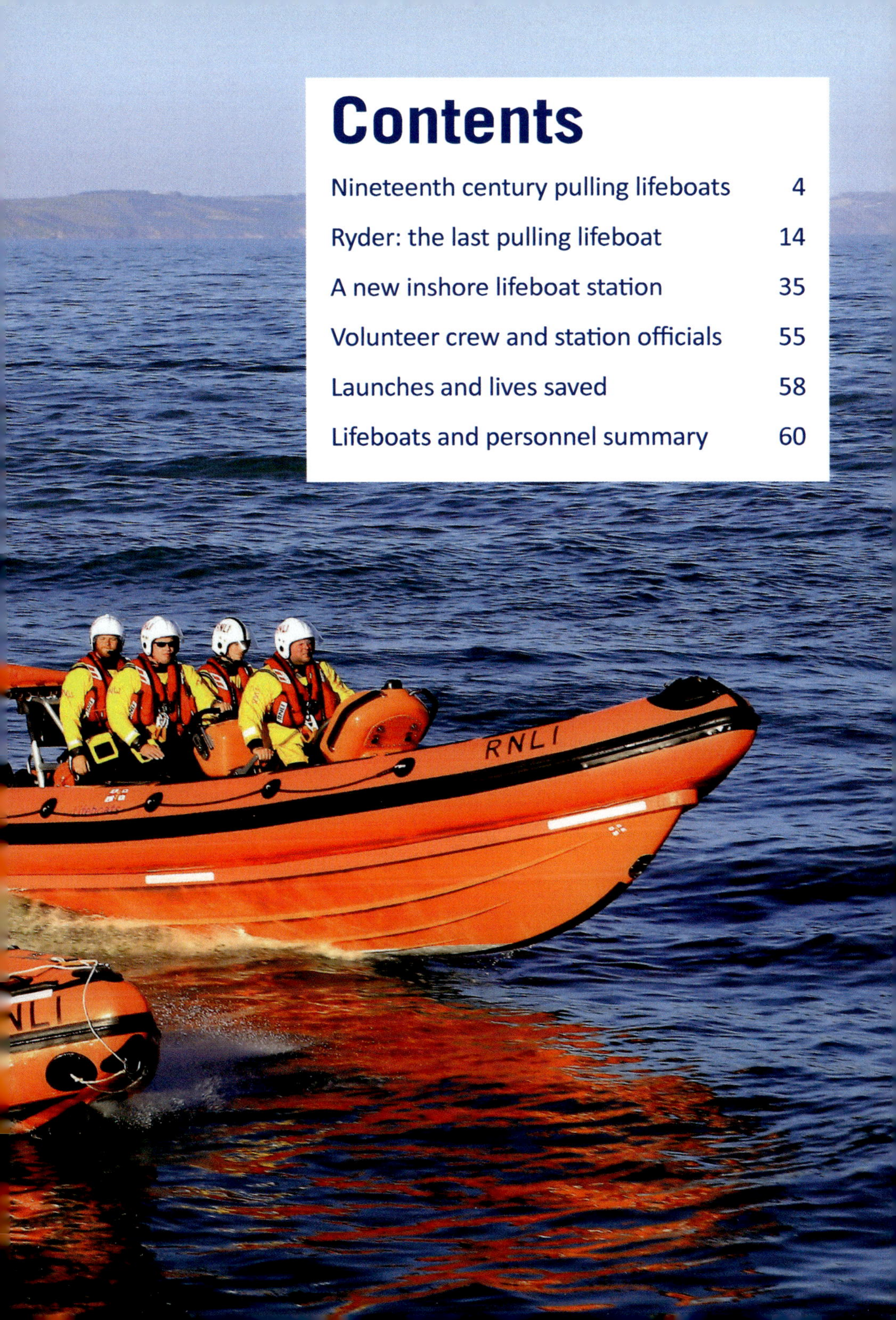

1866 – 1902
NINETEENTH CENTURY PULLING LIFEBOATS

The ancient seaport of Looe is situated on the south-east coast of Cornwall, at the head of a bay and in the mouth of a river which both share its name. The town is divided by a river into an East and West part, and each once formed a distinct borough returning members to Parliament. The place has a long and colourful history. It contributed as many as twenty ships and 315 men to the siege of Calais in the fourteenth century. The seamen of Looe have always shown courage in pursuing their hazardous vocation, and their record of lifesaving is a worthy one.

The lifeboat station at Looe was established in 1866 at a time when the Royal National Lifeboat Institution was expanding its operations throughout the country. The second half of the nineteenth century was the heyday of the 'standard' self-righting lifeboat, which had been perfected since its conception in 1851 so that by the 1880s it was almost the only type

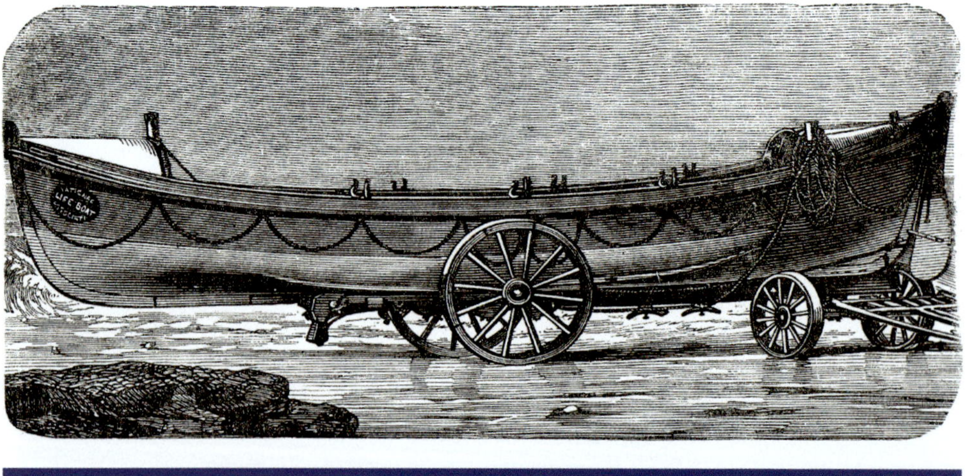

▼ A generic illustration of the RNLI's standard self-righter of the late nineteenth century. Looe's first lifeboat was similar in appearance.

of lifeboat in use. The self-righter was primarily a rowing boat, 34ft or 35ft in length, usually pulled by ten oars, and its radius of action was rather limited, although later boats carried sails. For this reason, the stations where they were operated were often in close proximity to one another so that the danger spots were adequately covered. The three pulling lifeboats that served Looe from 1866 until its closure in 1930 were all self-righters.

Frequent wrecks

Wrecks had not been infrequent in the Looe area prior to the opening of the lifeboat station. Vessels were often unable to round Rame Head to reach the safety of Plymouth Sound in heavy weather and took shelter in Whitsand Bay, to the east of Looe. In days of sail there was also a regular trade into and out of Looe River and, when the wind was from the south-east, entering the harbour could be both dangerous and difficult. Prior to the founding of the lifeboat station, several rescues were carried out at Looe by the Coastguard and local volunteers.

One came in the early hours of 23 November 1824, when the Dutch brig *Harmonie*, bound from Surinam for Hamburg, was driven ashore at Polorn Cove in heavy seas and six members of her crew were lost. The Coastguard heard cries for help and, led by Chief Boatman to the Coastguard, John Miller, a team of Coastguards made for the spot. In the darkness, they managed to climb down the cliffs to the wreck and rescued the remaining seven members of the ship's crew. For his gallantry and leadership on this occasion, John Miller was awarded a Silver medal by the RNLI.

In very heavy seas and a full gale, on 27 November 1838, the brig *Belissima*, of London, was driven onto rocks close to Looe Island, and the local coastguard attended the scene. As the brig began to break up, William Jennings, Commissioned Boatman with the Coastguard at Looe, volunteered to swim to the wreck, taking a line with him. A strong swimmer, Jennings battled pounding waves to reach the vessel and the crew of thirteen men were rescued. For his outstanding gallantry, Jennings was awarded a Silver Medal by the RNLI.

Another early rescue took place late on the evening of 14 February 1851 after the French brig *Fletan* was driven ashore in Whitsand Bay. The wreck was not spotted until next morning, when Chief Officer at Stoke Coastguard Station, John Anderson, with a team of Coastguards, hurried to the scene. Despite heavy seas pounding on the beach, Anderson and Richard Andrew waded out up to their shoulders in the water to get a rope on board the brig. Using this, the Coastguard managed to save the entire crew of nine men. For his gallantry, Anderson was awarded a Silver medal by the RNLI.

Founding the station

Further shipwrecks occurred in the area in the 1860s. The ship *Renovatio* was lost with all hands in 1865, and this demonstrated the need for a lifeboat and provided the impetus for the establishment of a station at Looe. The matter was raised with the RNLI in the spring of 1866 when, at a meeting of the RNLI's Committee of Management on 5 April, a letter from local residents was presented regarding the provision of a rescue craft; they suggested a Coastguard type lifeboat, or a 'whale-boat', be supplied. However, the RNLI's Committee stated, 'it would be better to have a proper lifeboat', and set about establishing a new lifeboat station. It was recommended to the people of Looe that the RNLI would provide a standard self-righting lifeboat, and this was accepted by the residents.

On 1 May 1866 the RNLI's Inspector of Lifeboats, Captain John Ward, RN, visited the area,

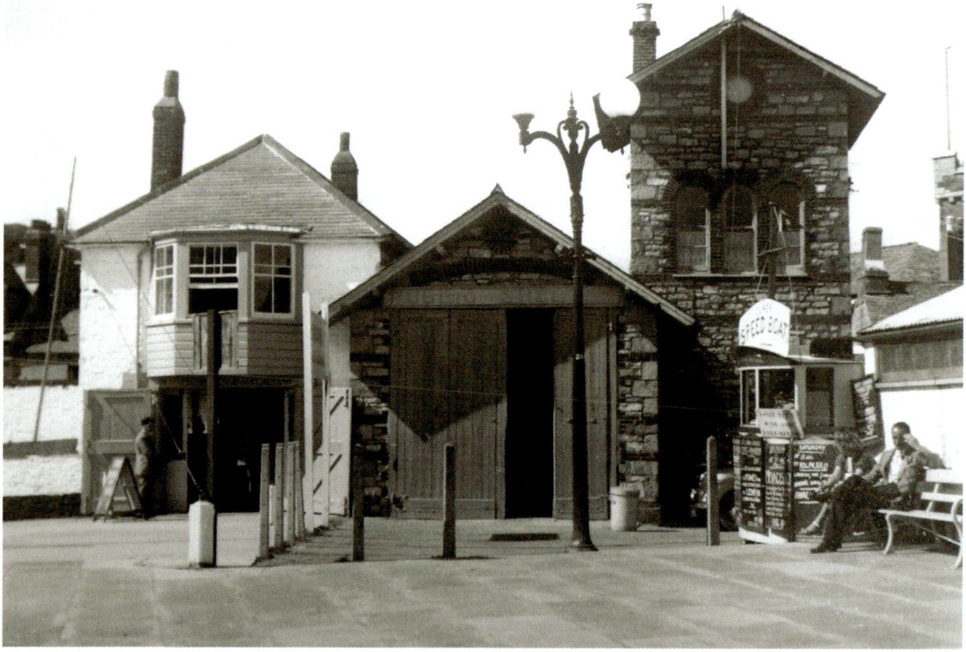

▲ When the station was established, the lifeboat house was built close to the harbour at East Looe, facing the beach, by local builders Sargent & Auger, and cost £220. Because of its prominent position, it was given an unusual ornamental design, with a reading and assembly room above the boathall for the use of local pilots and fishermen. In practice, the lifeboatmen used the lower part of the tower for storing their equipment, such as oilskins, rockets and so on, while the upper storey served as a committee room and lookout. The original lifeboat house lasted throughout the life of the station, and is still in existence. In June 1951, when this photograph was taken, the ground floor was being used as a public shelter with the lifeboat record boards on the walls. (Grahame Farr, by courtesy of the RNLI)

New lifeboat stations in Cornwall

No fewer than ten new stations were established by the RNLI in Cornwall between 1865 and 1885, and all were supplied with self-righting lifeboats. On the south coast, as well as Looe, new stations were opened at Falmouth, Cadgwith and Mullion (all 1867); Mevagissey and Porthoustock (both 1869); Portloe (1870); and a No.2 station was opened at Lizard (1885). On the north coast, lifeboats were placed at Hayle (1866) and Port Isaac (1869).

to assess the situation and select a site suitable for a boathouse. He also recommended a 32ft ten-oared 'medium lifeboat with transporting carriage' be ordered. Funding for the new station came from Sir John Pollard Willoughby, a civil servant and politician from Oxfordshire, who, on 24 March 1866, forwarded £420 to the RNLI. The money had been raised among various residents in his native county for providing a lifeboat to be named *Oxfordshire*, and it was appropriated to the new station. Meanwhile, the Mayor of Looe, Mr Bishop, said that he believed £200 could be raised locally towards the cost of the house, and work on the new building began towards the end of the summer.

The station's first lifeboat was a standard 32ft by 7ft 6in ten-oared self-righting type, built by Woolfe, at Shadwell in London, one of the RNLI's regular boatbuilders of this period, at a cost of £247 15s 0d. She was provided with a launching carriage, which cost a further £84 19s 6d. The lifeboat successfully passed her harbour trial on 21 December 1866, and everything was ready by the following day to get the boat to her station. Together with her gear, she was forwarded from London by rail. The GWR, the Bristol and Exeter, the South Devon and the Cornwall Railway Companies all provided free carriage for the new lifeboat, which eventually reached Liskeard railway station on 28 December 1866.

Upon arrival at Liskeard, she was placed on her carriage and drawn to Looe by a team of ten horses. On reaching the town, however, the narrow streets caused difficulties. One mast struck a shop near the

Oxfordshire services

1867	Jan 5	Fishing boat *Emelyne*, of Plymouth, no effective service
1867	Dec 1	Schooner St *Branock*, of Bideford, assisted to refloat vessel
	2	Unknown schooner, rounding Rame Head, no service
1868	Mar 27	Fishing boat, of Looe, saved boat and 2
	Sep 25	Schooner *Elizabeth Devy*, of Goole, assisted to save vessel and 3
	Dec 14	Schooner *Mail*, of Alloa, assisted to save vessel and 6
1869	Feb 4	Unknown barque, services not required
1873	Jan 9	Unknown vessel, no service
1874	Dec 8	Schooner *Carolina*, of Amsterdam, stood by
1876	Sep 30	Lugger *Jane Foster*, no service
1880	Oct 22	Fishing boat *Ada*, of Devonport, moored boat and saved 2
1881	Aug 29	Ketch *Lion*, of Exeter, saved 1

entrance to Fore Street, and as the street became ever narrower the carriage pulled off the water-spout of a house. The boat was then taken off her carriage and proceeded on runnels to the beach. The carriage followed, and the boat was placed on it again in preparation for the inaugural ceremony, which took place that same day.

During the ceremony, Mrs Carew, wife of W.H. Pole-Carew, President of the Looe Branch of the RNLI, christened the lifeboat *Oxfordshire*. Robert Thomas was appointed Honorary Secretary, with William Alford as Coxswain and James Toms as Second Coxswain.

Oxfordshire served at Looe for sixteen years, during which time she launched fourteen times on service and saved fourteen lives and was, for the era, relatively busy. Her first service launch, on 5 January 1867, took place shortly after she had arrived at her station and involved her launching into a south-westerly gale. Rescues were most often undertaken when the wind was in this direction, while almost all of her services were to small trading ships or fishing vessels.

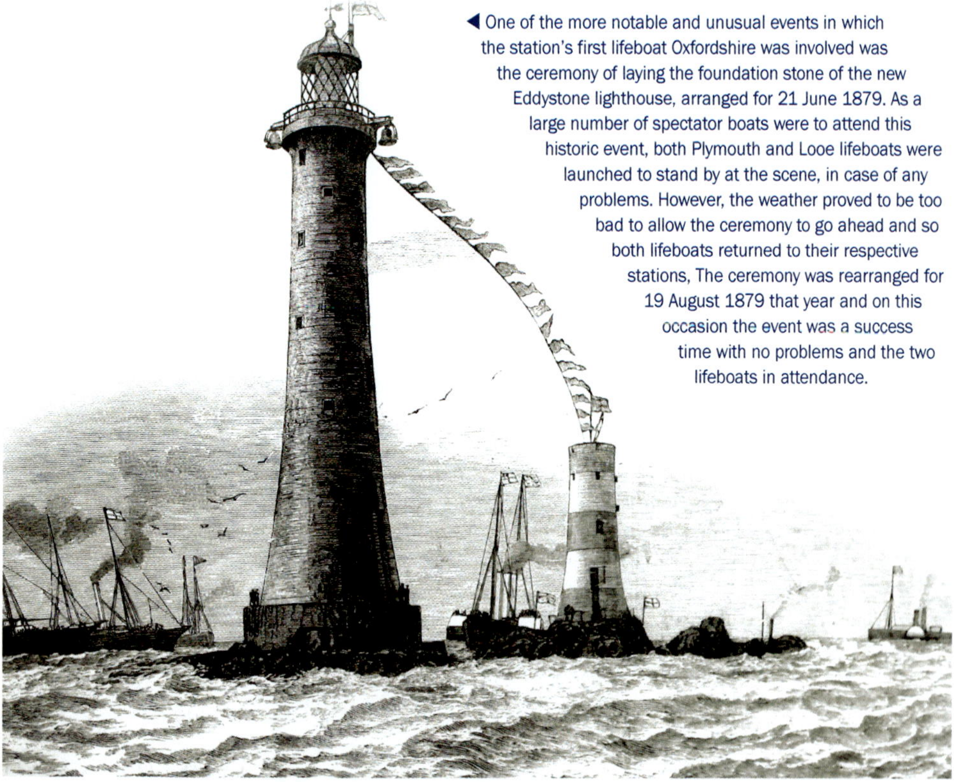

◀ One of the more notable and unusual events in which the station's first lifeboat Oxfordshire was involved was the ceremony of laying the foundation stone of the new Eddystone lighthouse, arranged for 21 June 1879. As a large number of spectator boats were to attend this historic event, both Plymouth and Looe lifeboats were launched to stand by at the scene, in case of any problems. However, the weather proved to be too bad to allow the ceremony to go ahead and so both lifeboats returned to their respective stations, The ceremony was rearranged for 19 August 1879 that year and on this occasion the event was a success time with no problems and the two lifeboats in attendance.

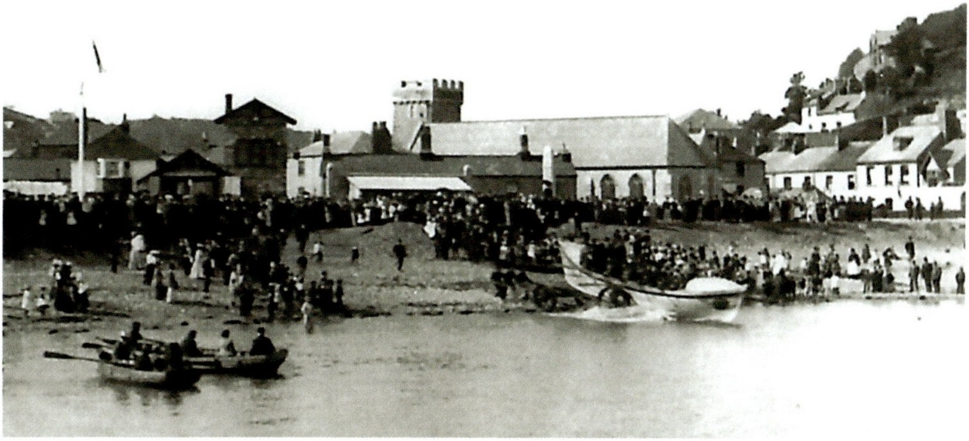

▲ The first Looe lifeboat Oxfordshire being launched off the beach, watched by a large crowd. It is believed this is the only photo of Oxfordshire, Looe's first lifeboat.

Boy's Own No.1

In February 1882 the RNLI decided, on the recommendation of the Chief Inspector, to replace *Oxfordshire*, which was then sixteen years old and an order was placed with Woolfe. The new lifeboat, 34ft ten-oared self-righter, was ready five months later, and on 13 July 1882 completed her harbour trial. Four days later the new boat and her carriage were forwarded to Cornwall by rail, being carried by the Great Western Railway Company, and the old boat and carriage were returned to London by the same route. On reaching Menheniot railway station, the boat was then placed on her carriage and taken to Looe.

The new lifeboat had cost £328 18s 0d, and its launching carriage £129. It was one of two new boats provided from funds raised by readers of the Boy's Own Paper, with the other going to Poole in Dorset; the Looe boat was named *Boy's Own No.1*, and the Poole boat *Boy's Own No.2*. A total of £600 had been received from the editor of the Paper, George A. Hutchinson, whose readers, mainly young and teenage boys, proved extremely generous in their support of the RNLI. The inauguration ceremony of the new boat took place on 21 July 1882, during which the Honorary Secretary reported that the boat 'had given satisfaction to the crew'.

Boy's Own No.1 served at Looe for twenty years, during which time she launched seven times on service and saved twenty-three lives. Her arrival was followed by a quiet period in the station's history and the new lifeboat did not undertake a service until 29 November 1888, more than six years after she arrived.

However, before her first service had been undertaken the lifeboat's self-righting abilities had been found wanting. On 23 December 1886 she had been taken out on exercise so that her self-righting qualities could be tested. She was deliberately capsized in the harbour in 12ft of water, but remained on her side until two of the crew clambered onto the keel and brought her round. The experiment was repeated twice, both times with similar unsatisfactory results. As a result, another lifeboat was sent to the station and the defective one withdrawn for further testing.

In January 1887 the District Inspector reported that he had tested the righting abilities of the temporary lifeboat, which were found to be fine. So *Boy's Own No.1* was taken away and alterations were made to the end boxes to give her a greater self-righting capability. This work took several months, and she did not return to Looe until July 1887 having been repaired and tested. Extra ballast had been fitted and, it was reported to the RNLI's Committee of Management, 'the results were very satisfactory'.

The service on 15 February 1900, to the ketch *Rib*, of Bridgwater, was the first with the lifeboat being launched from the Albatross slipway, which had been built to enable the boat to be launched into the river, and was for use mainly at low tide. Usually the lifeboat was taken over the beach on her carriage to be launched. The slip took its name from an old building which formed a quaint and picturesque architectural feature at Looe, and occupies more or less the same site as the slipway built for the inshore lifeboats.

The slipway was edged with rails to prevent the carriage slipping over the side, and its installation was an attempt to improve the launching arrangements, which had at times proved problematic. However, the

▼ The station's second pulling lifeboat, Boy's Own No.1, on her carriage, with her crew wearing their cork life-jackets. (By courtesy of Looe RNLI)

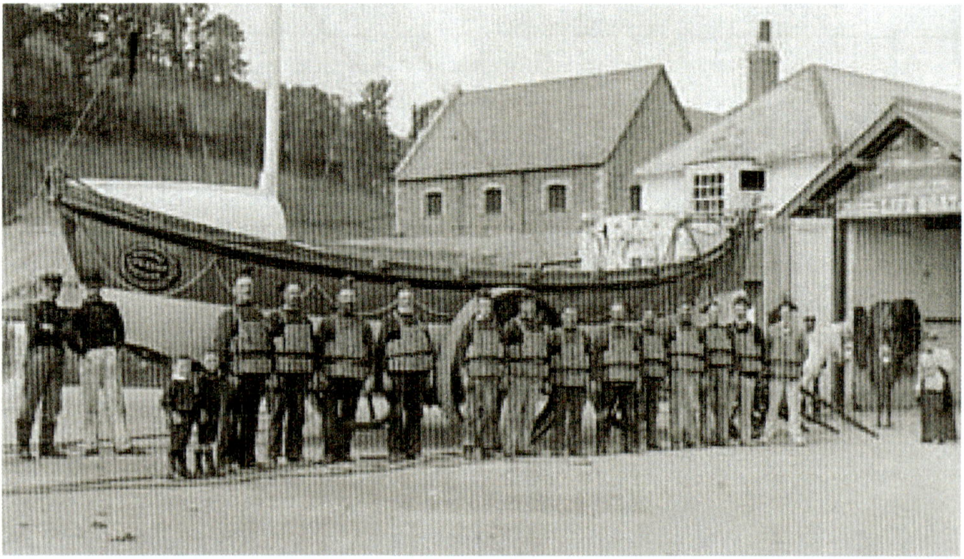

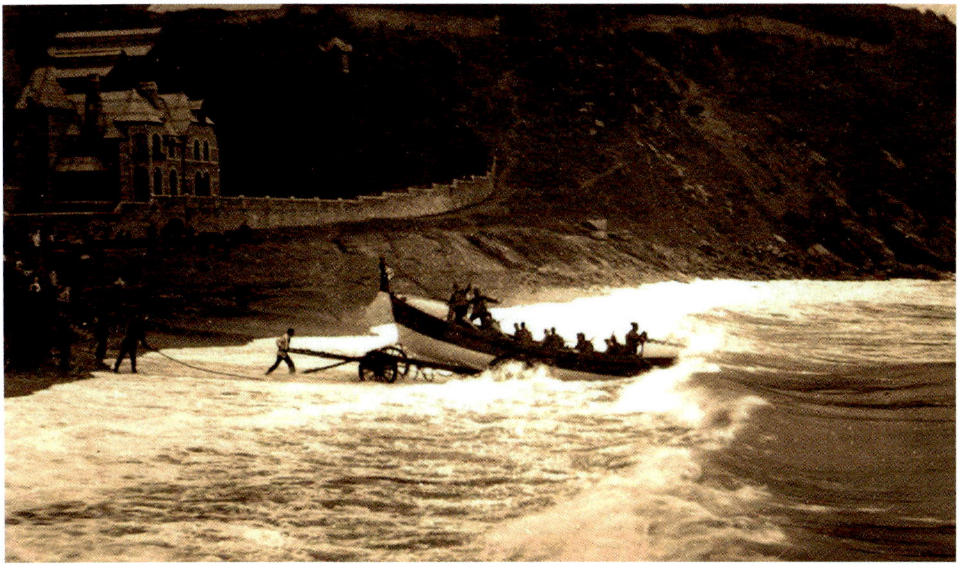

new slipway did not give complete satisfaction, for when the boat was launched on 28 December 1900, in response to rockets from the direction of the Eddystone, 'there was some delay in launching owing to the awkward construction of the slipway'. As a result, the boat's launch was delayed for more than an hour after the first rockets had been sighted. The wind being fair, sail was set and a course steered for the Eddystone, but nothing was found.

Service to ship Gipsy

The most noteworthy service carried out by the Looe lifeboat men with *Boy's Own No.1* took place on 7-8 December 1901, after the 1,447-ton full-rigged ship *Gipsy*, of Nantes, bound from Chile to Falmouth and Plymouth with a cargo of nitrates, lost her bearings. Mistaking the Downderry lights for those of Plymouth, she ran on rocks about 400 yards offshore from the Coastguard Station at Downderry. The volunteer crew assembled and an attempt was made to launch the lifeboat over the beach. But the front wheels of the carriage became embedded in the soft sand, and extra helpers were called, some of whom went into water up to their waists hauling on the boat to get her afloat. This resulted in some delay, but *Boy's Own No. 1* was eventually afloat at 6.30pm and proceeded under sail and oars to the wreck.

The lifeboat crew found the ship hard aground, and the captain asked that they fetch a tug. When told that a tug would be of no use, he said the lifeboat could return to her port, and he would signal by blue lights if he needed more help. Coxswain Edward Toms explained that the boat belonged to Looe,

▲ Boy's Own No.1 on being launched from East Looe beach on 21 July 1882. (By courtesy of Looe RNLI)

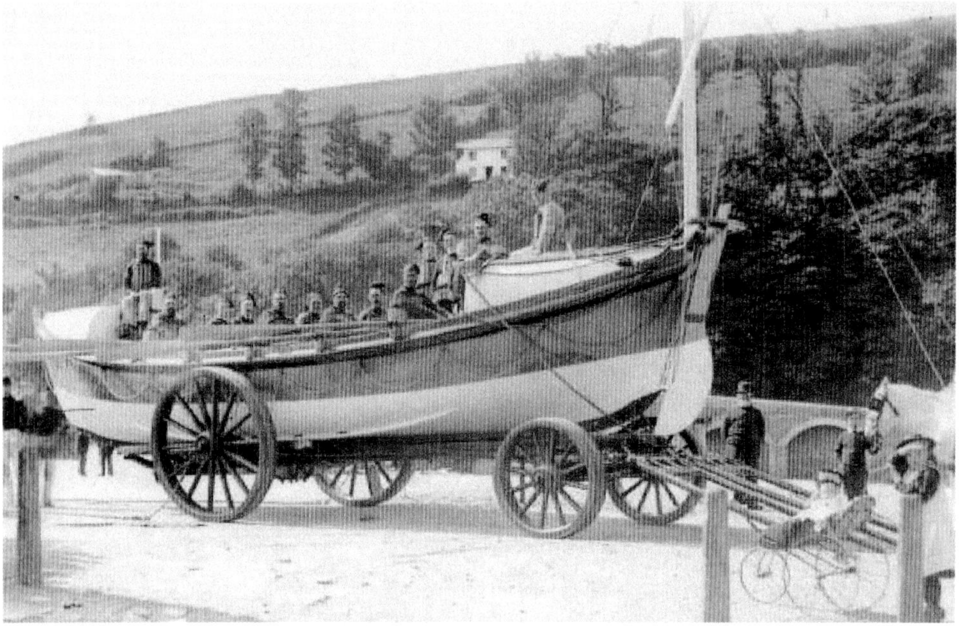

▲ Boy's Own No.1 on her launching carriage outside the boathouse. (By courtesy of Looe RNLI)

which was four miles distant, and eventually it was agreed that the lifeboat would stand by for a while. After trying, ineffectually, to pump out the water for two hours or more, the captain decided to abandon ship. Accordingly fourteen of his crew were taken aboard *Boy's Own No.1*, and the remaining five took to the ship's own boat, which was then taken in tow by the lifeboat.

Progress was very slow as the wind was rapidly rising and the sea was worsening; but when about halfway home, the lifeboat crew saw a tug and the lifeboat showed a red light for assistance. The tug was soon on scene and took the boats in

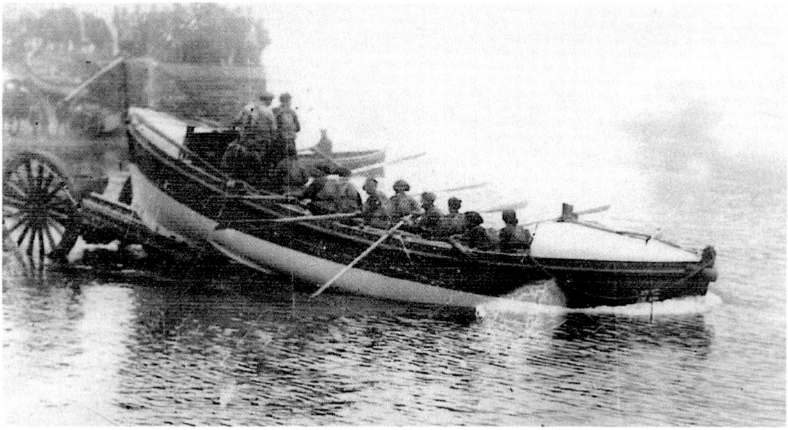

▶ Boy's Own No.1 being launched from the Albatros slipway into the river. (By courtesy of Looe RNLI)

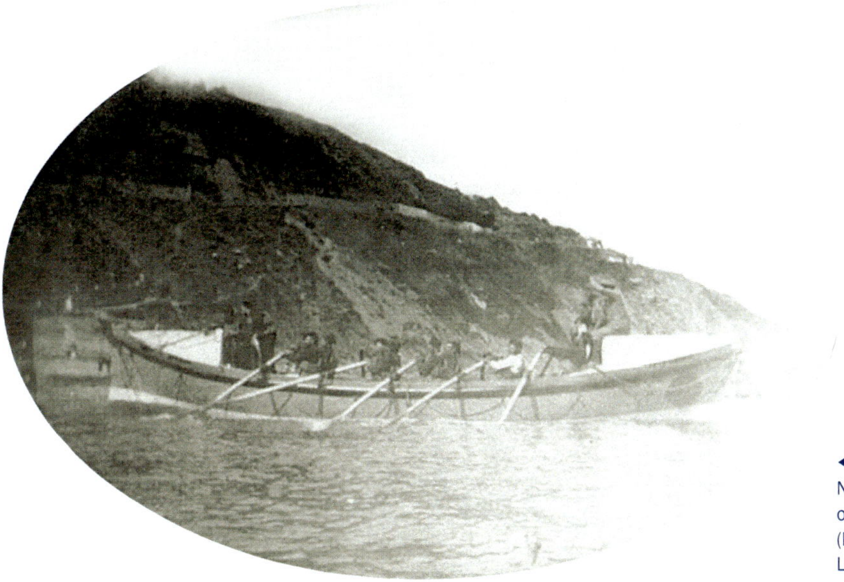

◀ Boy's Own No.1 under oars off Looe beach. (By courtesy of Looe RNLI)

tow; they arrived safely at Looe at 1.30am the following day. The ship remained stuck on the rocks and had become a total loss by daybreak.

In May 1902 the Board of Trade sent a letter to the RNLI stating that, in recognition of this fine rescue, the French Government had awarded a Gold Medal, Second Class, to Coxswain Edward Toms, and Silver Medals, Second Class, to each of the crew, Second Coxswain Percy Pearn, Bowman Joseph Fletcher, Thomas Toms, Robert Whynall, Ben Menhenick, Charles Toms, Ben Pengelly, Ernest Bettison, Albert Bettison, Francis Taylor, Thomas Pengelly and Stephen Cox, with Diplomas also being presented.

Replaced

By the time of this service, *Boy's Own No.1* had been found to be defective. In March 1901 the District Inspector reported that her water ballast tanks had not dried out and that the ventilation was inadequate. The air cases under the deck were also found to be in poor condition. The following month the local committee stated that the nineteen-year-old lifeboat should be replaced by 'a more modern type'. The RNLI's Committee were readily in agreement with this assessment, and the process of providing a new lifeboat got under way.

Boy's Own No.1 services

1888	Nov 29	Barquentine *St Halvard*, of Plymouth, no service rendered
1894	Jan 9	Trawler *Louie*, of Brixham, no service
1897	Dec 2	Ketch *Foundling*, of Brixham, stood by
1900	Feb 13	Six crab boats, of Looe, escorted over bar
	15	Ketch *R.T.B.*, of Bridgwater, saved 4
	Dec 28	Unknown vessel, no service
1901	Dec 7	Ship *Gipsy*, of Nantes, saved (also 3 kittens) 19

1902 –1930

RYDER: THE LAST PULLING LIFEBOAT

▼ Ryder on her carriage being hauled down the Albatross slipway to be launched.

When assessing the most suitable new boat for Looe, the Coxswain and crew considered that one with a drop keel would be best suited to the station's needs. After they had visited other stations to examine lifeboats at different locations, the local committee, coxswains and crew requested that a self-righting boat, 35ft by 8ft 6in, with slightly fallen lines forward, be built for Looe. The Coxswain also requested that the lifeboat was rigged with a dipping lug, as all the boats in Looe were rigged this way, and the fishermen, who would form the crew, would be familiar with this set up. The RNLI agreed to this request and ordered a lifeboat from Thames Ironworks,

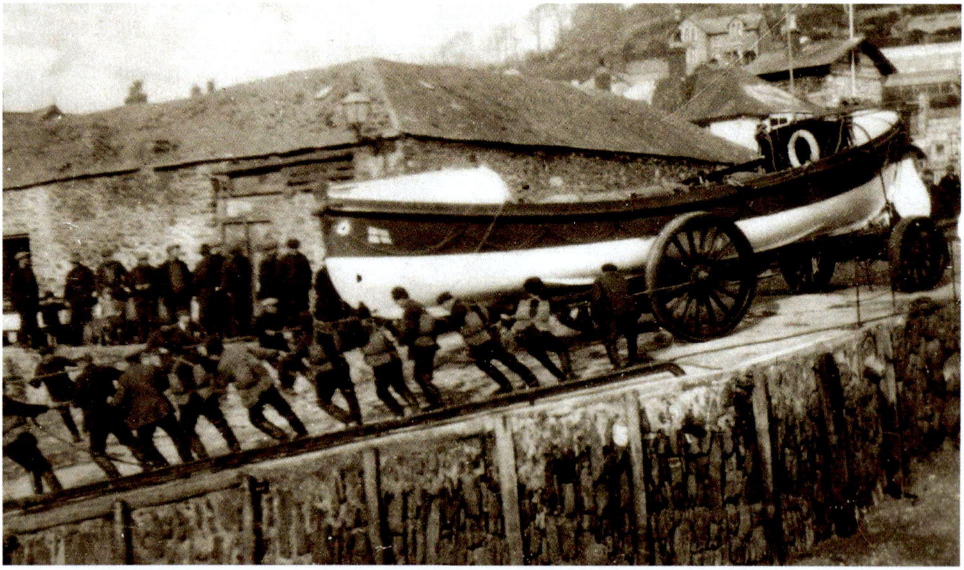

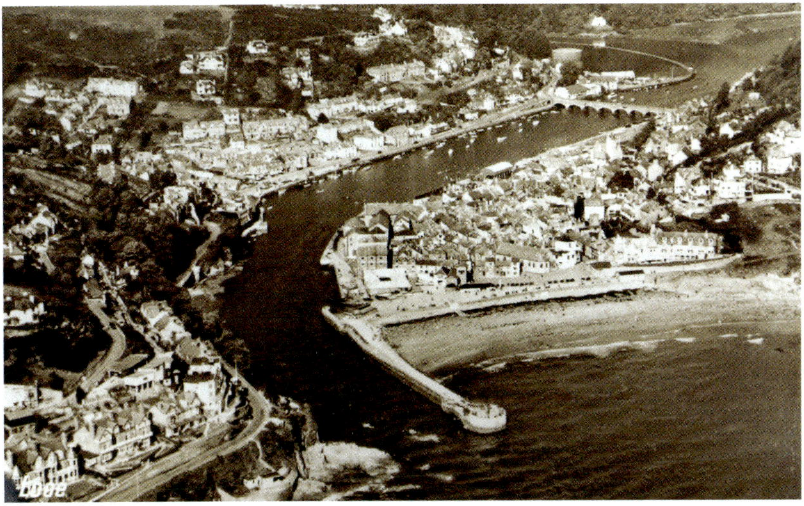

◀ An aerial view of Looe town, river and harbour, with the original lifeboat house lower centre.

of Blackwall, the boatyard where more than 100 lifeboats were built during the late nineteenth and early twentieth centuries.

Funds for the new boat came from a legacy of £1,500 bequeathed to the RNLI by the late William Ryder of Brixton Road, London, to provide a lifeboat named *Ryder*. This money was appropriated to the Looe boat in July 1901.

It took almost a year for the new lifeboat to be completed, but on 22 May 1902 she passed her trials on the Thames and was ready for service. Arrangements were made to transport her to Cornwall, and on 25 May she was sent by railway to Plymouth, with the Great Western Railway providing free carriage, and from there she was taken by sea to Looe, being sailed to her new station by some of her crew. The old lifeboat and carriage were sold locally, as was the usual practice at the time.

Ryder was a 35ft self-righter, as the crew had requested, pulled ten oars, had a dipping lug and mizen, and was fitted with a 10ft keel with a 2ft drop so that she could be taken out under sail. She served at Looe for almost three decades, becoming the longest serving as well as the last of the station's pulling lifeboats. She was launched on service twelve times and saved thirty-seven lives. Descriptions are included below of her most notable rescues.

The first service performed by *Ryder* was undertaken in the early hours of 27 February 1903. She launched at 2.40am to the 575-ton steamer *Daisy*, of Liverpool, and was out for almost three hours in the darkness helping the steamer's crew. The next services took place during the afternoon of 10 September 1903, when she helped the smack *William*, of Par. Within an hour of landing the smack's two crew, the lifeboat was called out again.

Having been left afloat in the

harbour, she was quickly manned and put to sea, going to the aid of the local lugger *Anemone*, which, with a crew of four, was drifting towards the shore in heavy seas having lost most of her sails in the storm. *Ryder* reached the vessel when she was within half-a-mile of the shore, and was taken alongside. The lifeboat men saved two of the lugger's crew before the lifeboat was swept clear. Coxswain Toms then skilfully manoeuvred the lifeboat back into position so the remaining two men could be rescued, by which time the gale had risen to hurricane force. The survivors were landed at the station at 7.30pm.

The RNLI granted additional financial rewards to each of the lifeboat crew involved in this excellent service. They were: Coxswain Edward Toms, Second Coxswain Percy Pearn, Bowman Thomas Toms, and Francis Taylor, Stephen Cox, Edward Pearn, Thomas Pengelly, Edward Pengelly, Richard Stephens, Charles Symons, Harry Symons, Samuel Symons and Charles Hocking.

Launching the lifeboat at Looe had been difficult at times, and shortly after *Ryder* had arrived on station discussions were held about how to improve matters. In February 1902 the District Inspector and honorary secretary pointed out that the lifeboat could not be transported by road, as was possible at many stations, and that the carriage could only be used for the launching the lifeboat opposite

▼ With launchers ready at the ropes, Ryder is brought out of her boathouse watched by a good crowd of locals and visitors. (By courtesy of Looe RNLI)

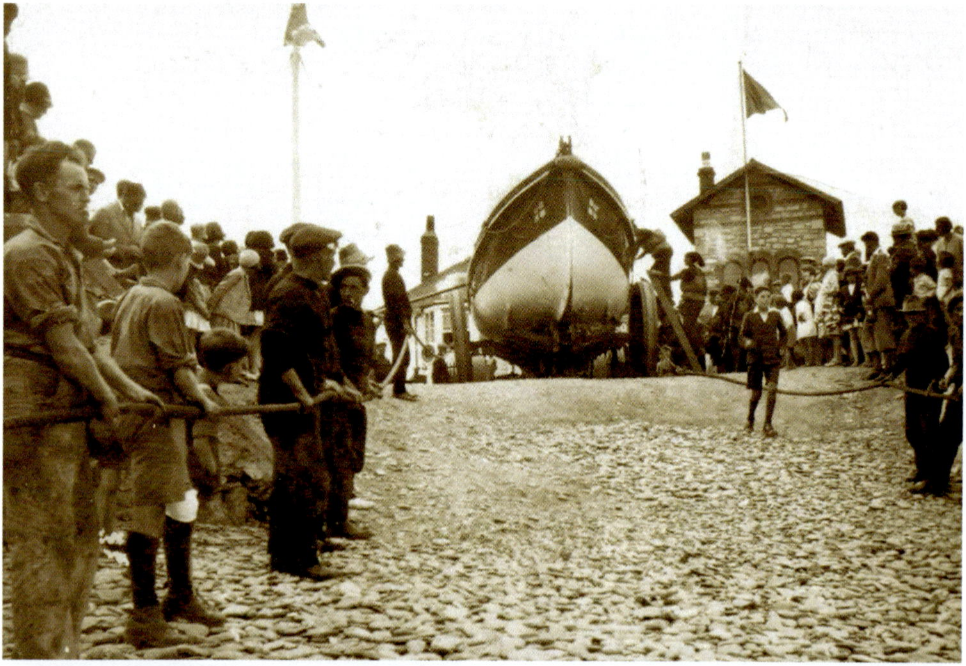

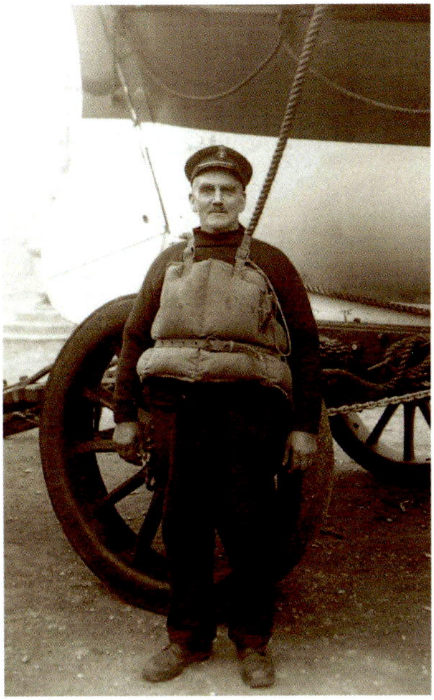

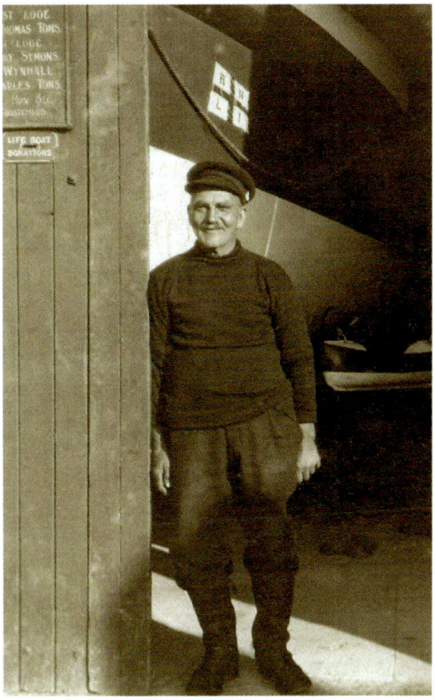

◀ Two photos of Coxswain Thomas Toms, standing in front of the lifeboat wearing his kapok life-jacket, circa 1928 (on left), and in front of Ryder. Toms, the former bowman, was the last Coxswain of the pulling lifeboats, serving in the post from 1919 to 1930. The former bowman, he took over as coxswain when Edward Toms retired. When the station was closed in July 1930, Thomas Toms was one month short of his 70th birthday.

the boathouse, either into the river or off the beach.

The Chief Inspector therefore recommended that the new carriage that had been built for the lifeboat be appropriated elsewhere, and a carriage from the Nairn station in Scotland be prepared for Looe. Although there is no further information about these carriages, presumably the new one originally built for *Ryder* was intended to be used on the road, to take the lifeboat to different launch sites.

In January 1903 further difficulties with launching were experienced, when it was reported that lowering the carriage down the slipway into the river was a dangerous operation. As the slipway was the property of the harbour commissioners, making alterations to it required their permission. A small temporary curb was built on the south side of the slip to stop the lifeboat's carriage slipping off.

But the problems continued, and in May 1903 attention was again called to the difficulty and possible danger of lowering the lifeboat on her carriage down the harbour slip on a dark night, between half ebb and half flood. The RNLI's Chief Inspector recommended that, as the house was cramped and deemed to be unsuitable, the RNLI's Architect report on the slipway and also assess whether any alterations to the house were necessary.

A couple of months after his visit, the Architect stated that both the house and slipway should be removed and new ones constructed. He estimated the cost of a new

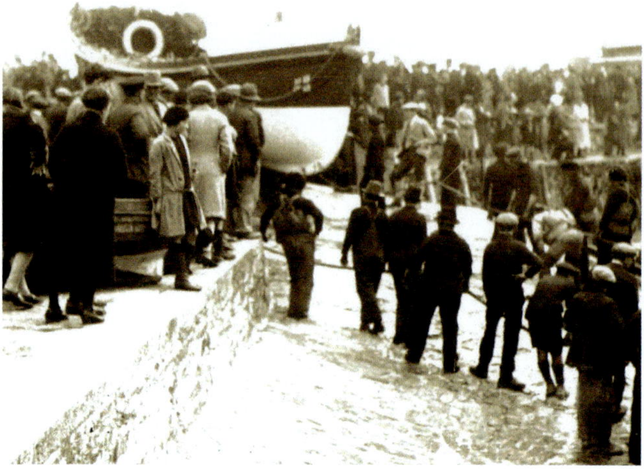

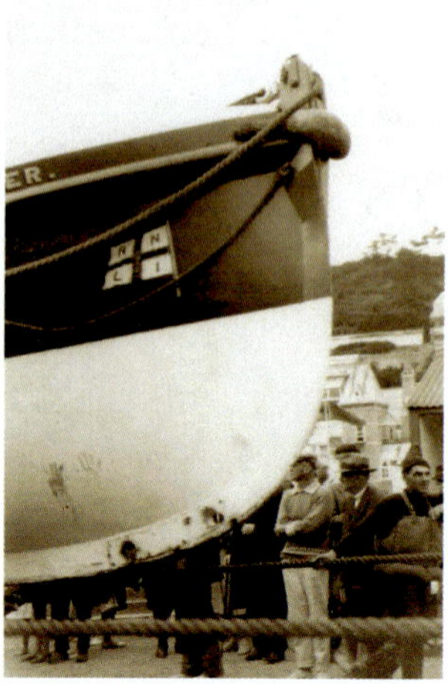

▲ Ryder being launched into the river via the Albatross slipway, with a good crowd watching the spectacle.

house at £800 and a slipway at £425. The additional ground for a new house would have to be obtained from the East Looe Harbour Trust and the permission of the harbour board would be required to construct a new slipway. When taking this into account, he suggested that moving the station to a completely different site might in fact be preferable. A deepwater launching site could be obtained on the west side of the harbour and outside the bar.

The problems of launching were again highlighted after the Deputy Chief Inspector witnessed a launch at dead low-water spring tide in October 1903 which took half an hour. He discussed with the local committee how the launching arrangements could be improved, but representatives of the harbour trustees said that the intended expansion of the slipway would not be approved by the harbour board.

The local committee were

The wreck of the French schooner St Pierre, February 1906. The lifeboat, under Coxswain Edward Toms, was launched from the beach though a very heavy sea. The Coxswain handled the boat in 'a masterly manner' and took her alongside the casualty, quickly effecting the rescue of her five crew, and Ryder and her crew were back in a little over an hour. ▶

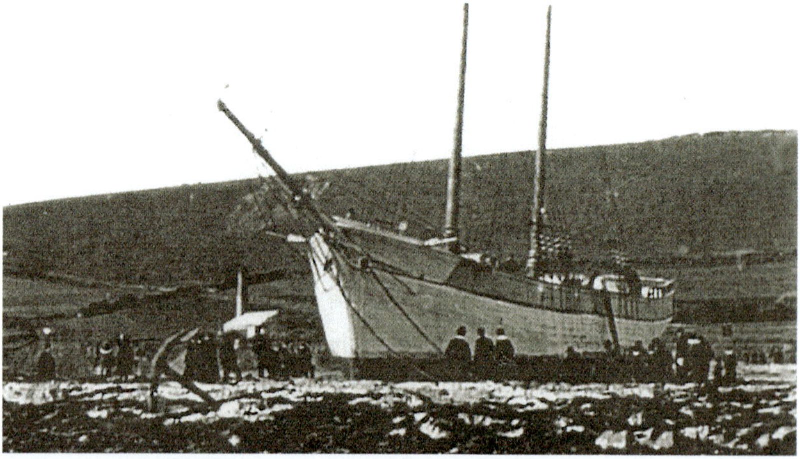

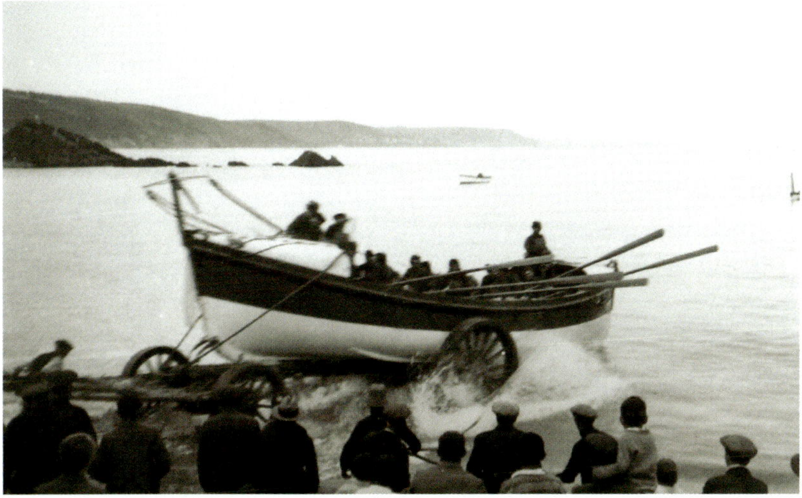

◀ With the carriage entering the water, Ryder is launched across the beach. (By courtesy of Looe RNLI)

unanimously in favour of moving the station to West Looe to a site on the Hannaford estate, which 'was in every way suitable for a boathouse and slipway to deliver the boat into deep water'. However, the RNLI could not justify such an expense as launching was possible most of the time. In the end, the Institution only considered it necessary for a haul-off warp to be installed for use at low water. In January 1904 repairs to the slipway were carried at a cost of £20, but after that the matter of a new boathouse and slipway, at a new site, was dropped and operations remained in the original house until the station closed.

The rescues undertaken by *Ryder* were relatively few and far between during her almost three decades of service. During the 1910s she was called out only a handful of times, and did not complete any life-saving services, although in June 1914 the District Inspector, when taking the boat out on exercise, concluded his report by stating that he 'had never seen such good oarsmen in a lifeboat before, except perhaps at Appledore', although no explanation was given as to what made Looe's or Appledore's crews so good.

The effective services undertaken by the Looe lifeboat crew in the 1920s were more notable, but none were spectacular. The first came on 3 March 1922, when she was launched at 6.30am after the Coastguard had reported that

▼ Ryder inside the lifeboat house on the sea front.

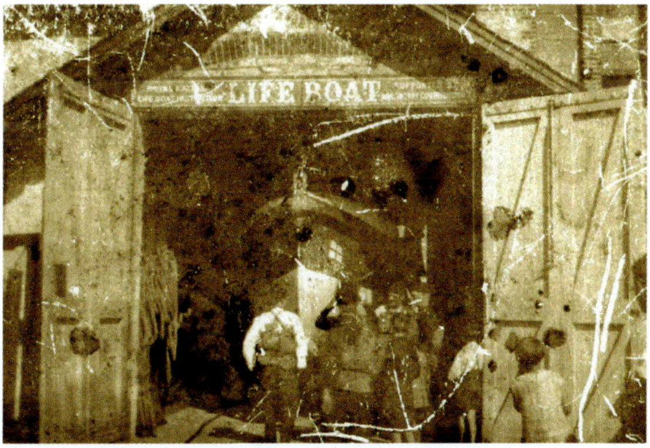

the 220-ton trawler *Marguerite*, of Boulogne, with a crew of twenty-one, had run aground just south of the Eddystone Reef, in rough seas and a strong south-westerly wind. But half an hour later news was received that, in fact, the trawler was aground in Talland Bay, just two miles west of Looe, and so signals were fired to recall the lifeboat. She was rowed and sailed back to Looe, where Coxswain Toms was given the latest position of the casualty.

The motor lugger *Dorothy* then towed the lifeboat to Talland Bay, where the lifeboat crew found the trawler hard aground, right in among the rocks, with heavy seas breaking over her. Coxswain Toms dropped anchor and the lifeboat was slowly veered down towards the vessel and, with a great deal of skill, was manoeuvred alongside. Although the wreck was being constantly swept by rough seas, the lifeboat rescued all twenty-one men, taking the master's young son on board first, and the master last. The trawler had about fifty tons of fish on board. The survivors were returned safely to Looe, being landed at 9.30am.

The next service took place on 27 May 1926 after the ninety-ton ketch *Zarita*, of Plymouth, with a crew of four, went aground on rocks near Looe Island during the afternoon. *Ryder* was launched at 4.40pm into rough seas and a very strong south-westerly wind. But, just as she came clear of her launching carriage, she was caught by a heavy sea and hit the carriage with sufficient force to put her steering gear out of action. But the lifeboat was afloat and the crew pulled at the oars to get her away from the beach. A local

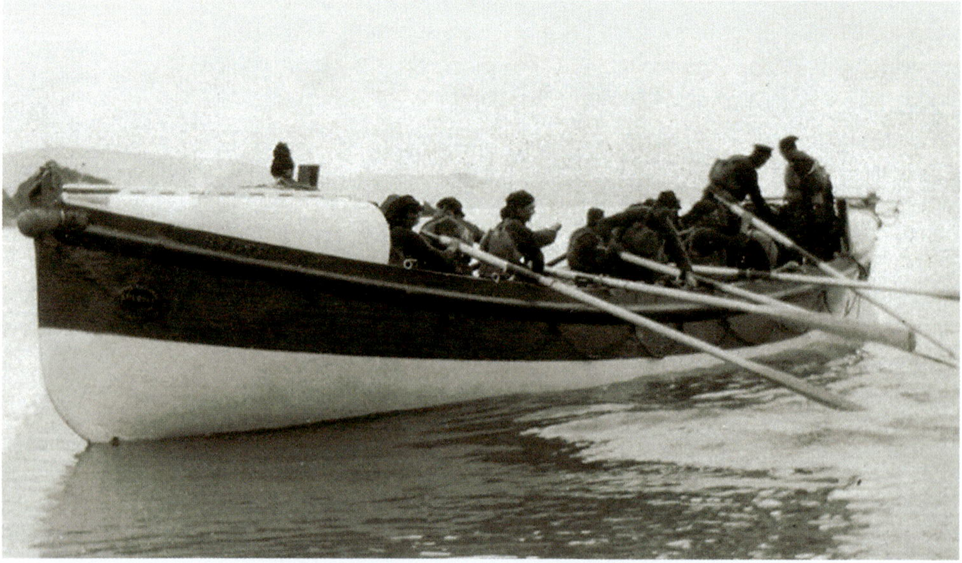

▼ Ryder being brought ashore under oars, ready to be recovered. After being beached, she would have been manhandled out of the water, and then hauled onto her carriage. (By courtesy of Looe RNLI)

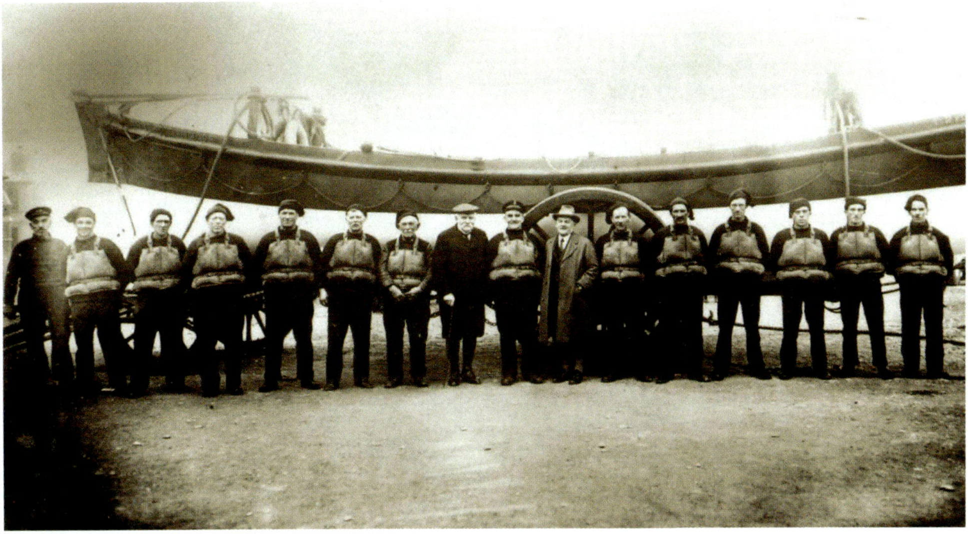

motor launch then took her in tow and headed to the accident, reaching the scene in just twenty minutes. The lifeboat was taken alongside the ketch and rescued three members of the crew, but the Master refused to leave, hoping to salvage his craft. However, as the tide began to rise, the ketch slowly filled with water and the lifeboat, which had stood by throughout, was taken alongside again and the master agreed to abandon ship. He was rescued, and the lifeboat then landed the four survivors at Looe at 7.15pm.

What proved to be *Ryder*'s last service took place on 18 April 1929. She was launched at 12.30pm after the large French liner *Paris*, with over 1,500 people on board and en route from Le Havre to New York, went aground on the Eddystone Reef in dense fog and a dead calm. The destroyer *Thanet*, dockyard tugs *Rover* and *Retort* from Plymouth, and the GWR tender *Sir Walter Raleigh* all went out to help.

Ryder and her crew were towed out by the motor launch *Our Girls*, the two boats quickly disappearing from the sight of those ashore in the fog. Fifteen minutes after setting

▲ Ryder on her carriage with the crew lined up in front of her, wearing their kapok life-jackets. (By courtesy of Looe RNLI)

Ryder services

1903	Feb 27	Steamship *Daisy*, of Liverpool, no service
	Sep 10	Smack *William*, of Par, saved 2
		Lugger *Anemone*, of Looe, saved 4
1906	Feb 22	Schooner *St Pierre*, of Nantes, saved 6
1911	Sep 10	Unknown vessel, no service
1913	Jan 14	Fishing boats, of Looe, escorted over bar
1914	June 20	Small boat, no service
1915	Feb 17	Steamship *Panama Transport*, of West Hartlepool, landed 6
1922	Mar 3	Trawler *Marguerite*, of Boulogne, saved 21
1923	Dec 7	Schooner *Mary Peers*, of Chester, no service
1926	May 27	Ketch yacht *Zarita*, of Plymouth, saved 4
1929	Apr 18	Steamship *Paris*, of Havre, no service

There is uncertainty about the exact number of lives saved by Ryder, 43 or 37; the issue is down to the six lives landed from the steamship Panama Transport, which were not classified as lives saved by the RNLI.

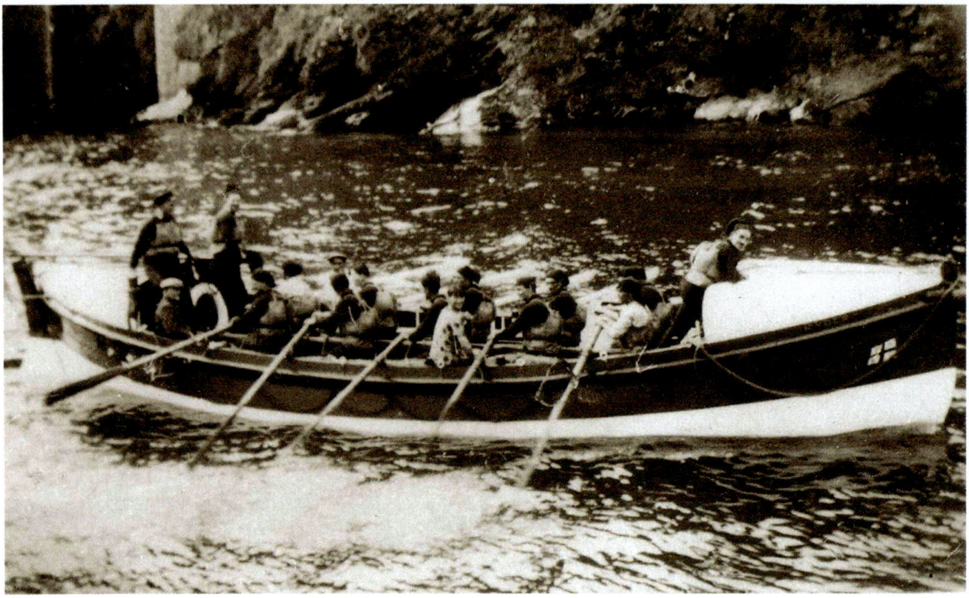

▲ Ryder under oars in Looe river, returning to station. This was the last quarterly exercise launch, in July 1930, before Ryder withdrawn from service. Mr Childs can be seen with a flat cap. (By courtesy of Looe RNLI

out, news was received at Looe that the liner had refloated and was making for Plymouth under her own power, and so recall signals were fired, but these were neither heard nor seen by the lifeboat crew, and so *Ryder* carried on to the Eddystone.

On reaching the reported position of the liner, the lifeboat men found no sign of her, with the lighthouse keepers informing Acting Coxswain Symons, the station's Second Coxswain, who was in command on this service, that the liner had refloated and gone to Plymouth. So the motor launch

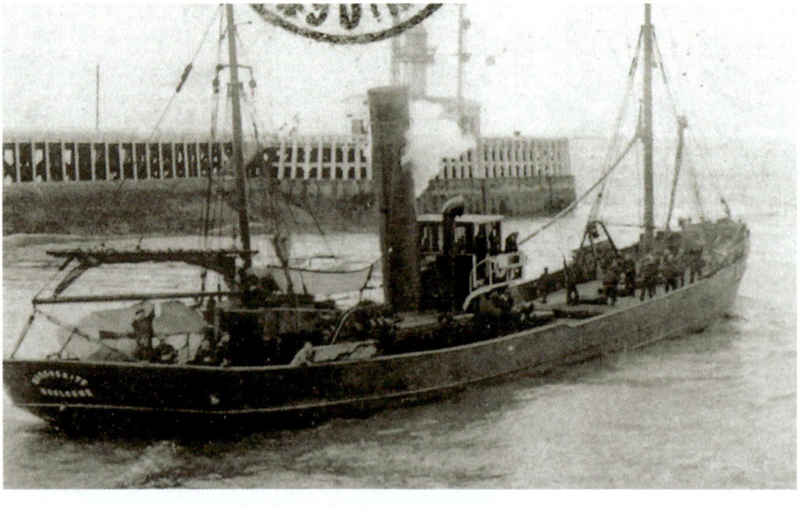

▶ The trawler Marguerite, of Boulogne, from which Ryder saved twenty-one people on 3 March 1922. (By courtesy of Looe RNLI)

towed the lifeboat back to Looe, and she arrived at her station at 5pm.

Closure of the station

By the time of the service to the liner, a large 60ft twin-engined Barnett motor lifeboat, named *Robert and Marcella Beck*, had been in service at Plymouth for three years, and in 1928 a motor lifeboat had been sent to Fowey. They could cover the area around Looe more effectively than the pulling lifeboat, and so, with the reduction in coastal sailing traffic also being taken into account, the RNLI, at a meeting of the Committee of Management on 10 April 1930, decided to close the Looe station. *Ryder* was duly withdrawn from service the on 30 July, and the lifeboat house was sold.

On the station's closure, William Thomas Toms, who had served as Coxswain for eleven and a half years and Second Coxswain for six and a half years, as well as being on the crew for many years, was granted an RNLI pension, and received a Certificate of Service.

Henry Symons, who, after several years as a member of the crew, had served as Bowman for more than six years and then as Second Coxswain for just over eleven years, was also granted a pension by the RNLI. Robert Wynhall, bowman for more than eleven years up to the station's closure, was also granted a pension, as was Charles Toms, who had been shore signalman for thirty-one and a half years. The station's service boards were later mounted to the wall of the old lifeboat house, which subsequently became a public shelter. In sixty-three years of service, the Looe lifeboat crews in the pulling lifeboats saved seventy-four lives and assisted

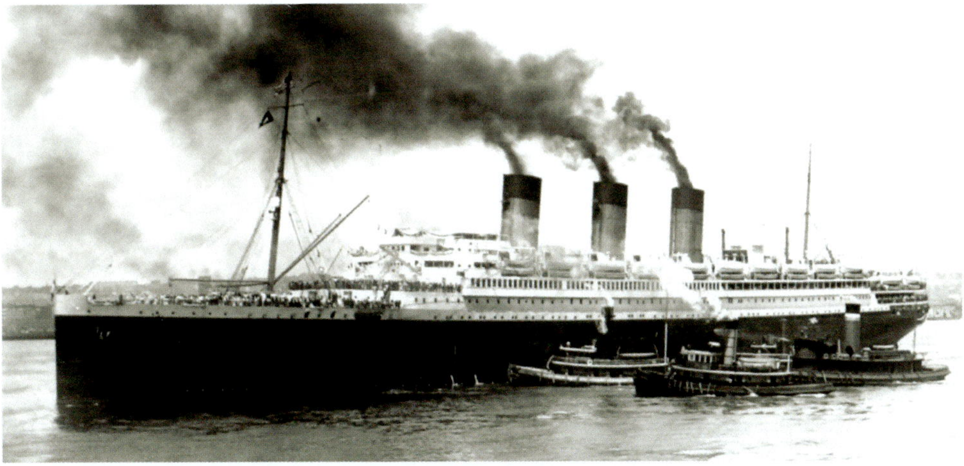

▲ The French liner Paris, built in Saint-Nazaire for the Compagnie Générale Transatlantique, being assisted into Plymouth by various tugs in April 1929 after she had struck the Eddystone Reef. When Paris was completed in the early 1920s, she was the largest liner under the French flag, at 34,569 tons, and was one of the most notable inter-war liners. (By courtesy of Looe RNLI)

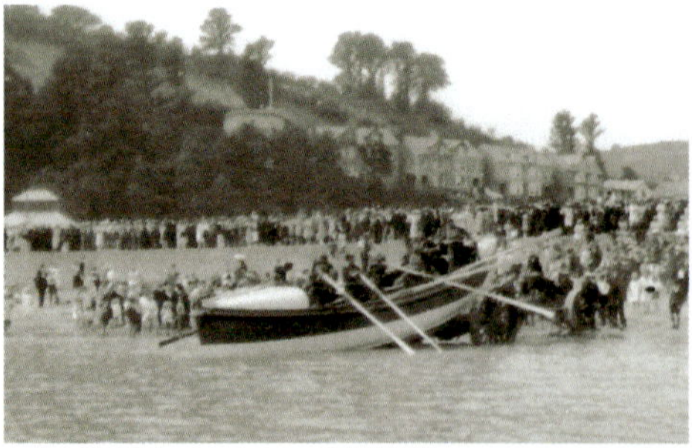

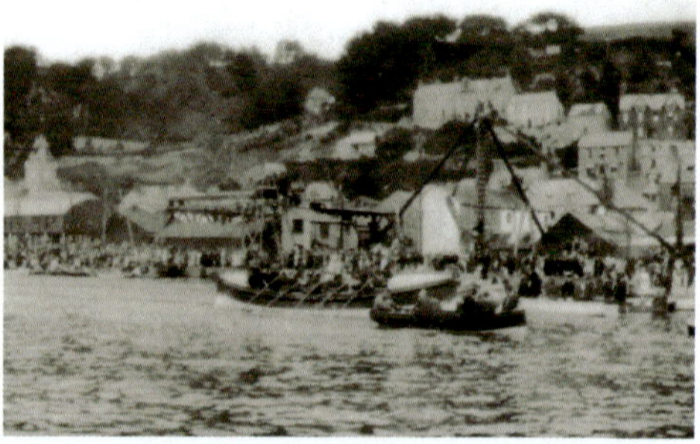

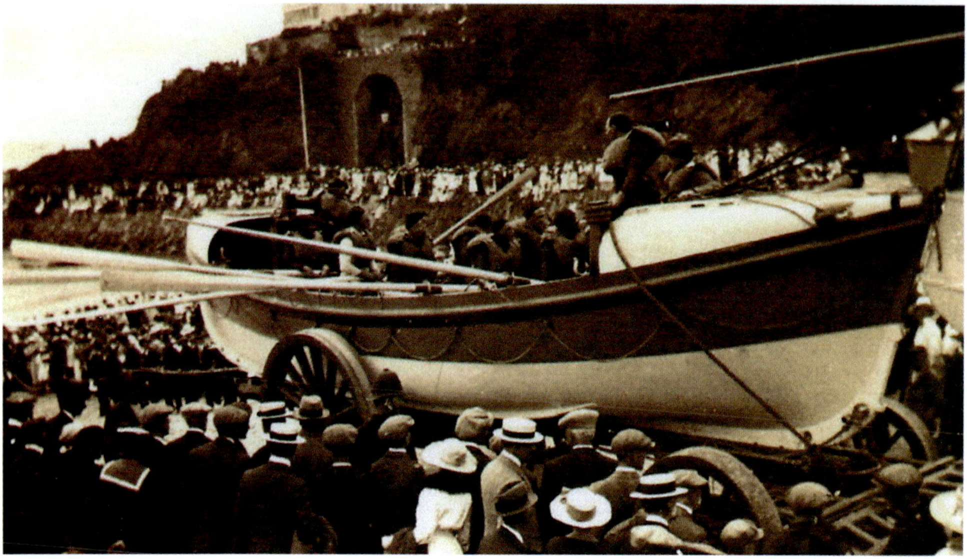

▲ Ryder being launched. (By courtesy of Looe RNLI)

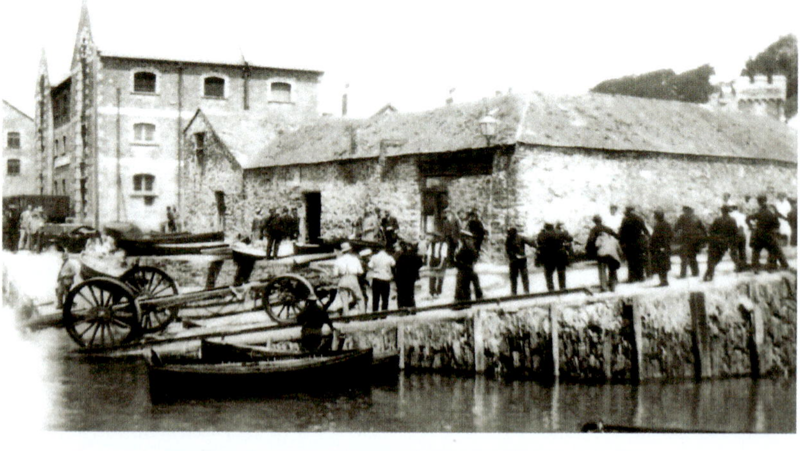

▶ The launching carriage is hauled back up the slipway after Ryder has been launched. (By courtesy of Looe RNLI)

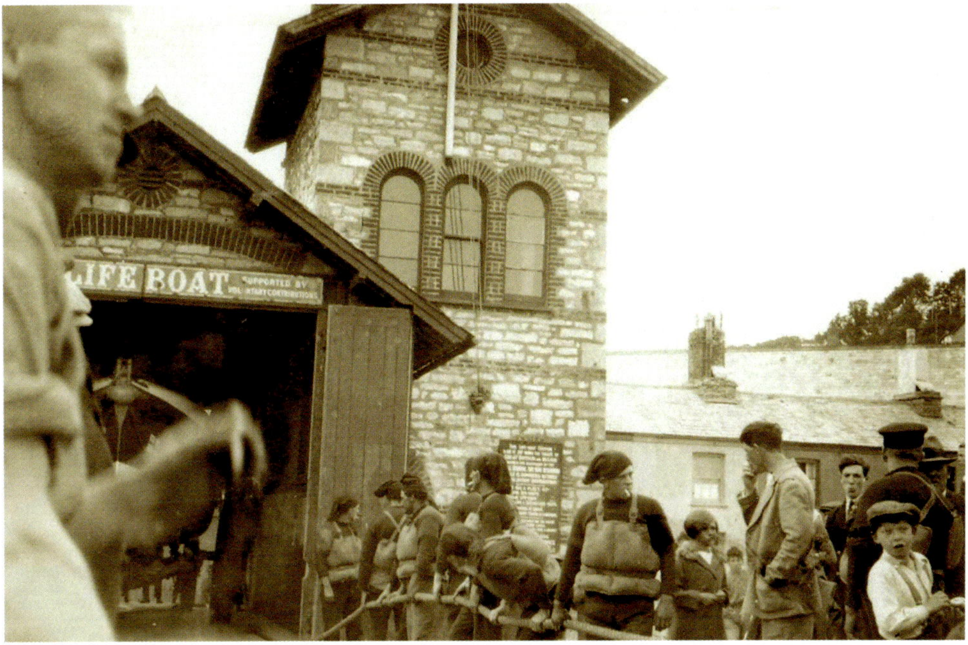

▲ The last launch of Ryder at Looe, July 1930, with the crew preparing to haul her out of the boathouse and take her to sea for the final time. (By courtesy of Looe RNLI)

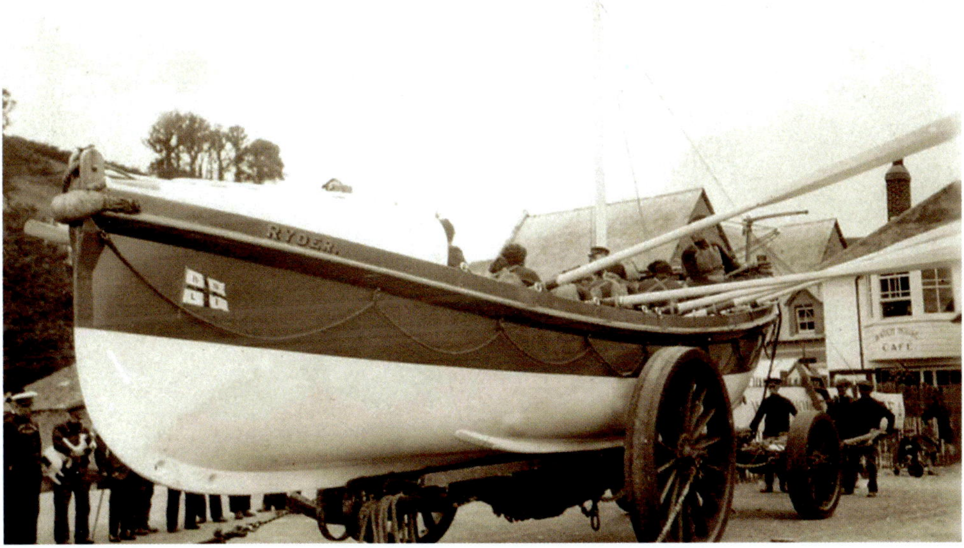

▲ The last demonstration launch of Ryder, with her crew at the oars for the final time, June 1930. (By courtesy of Looe RNLI)

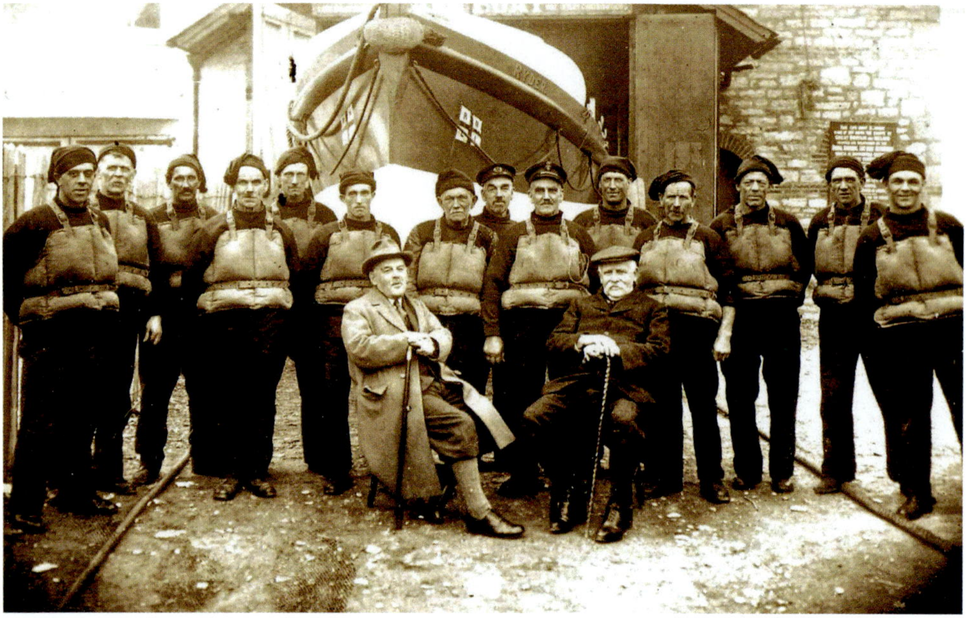

▲ The last crew of the pulling era, with Ryder on her carriage, 1928. They are, left to right: W. Butters, W. Cox, T. Cox, S. Symons, C. Hoskin, A. Hoskin, R. Wynhall, C. Toms (signalman), Thomas Toms (Coxswain), C. Hockin, H. Symons (Second Coxswain), R. Soady, C. Prynn and G. Soady; seated are W.F. Phillips (Honorary Secretary) and J. Child (Chairman). (Looe RNLI)

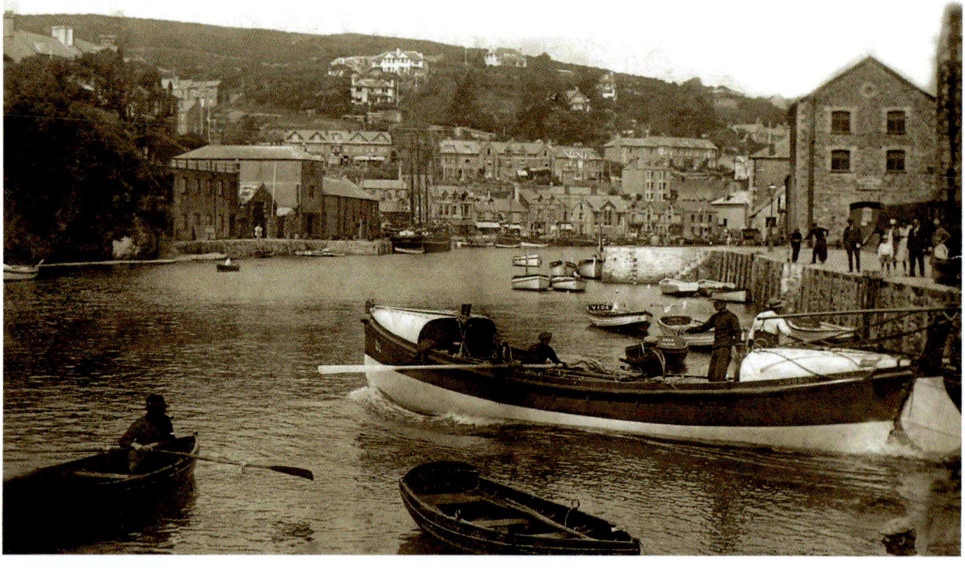

▲ Ryder being launched after her withdrawal and decommissioning from service to be taken to a mooring by the bridge. She has been stripped of equipment and grab lines. (By courtesy of Looe RNLI)

numerous vessels, notching up a creditable record.

Sold out of service

Although *Ryder* had ended her days as an operational lifeboat, she started a new life as the original one ended in July 1930. She was sold out of service to a Mr H. Taylor, of Rea Street in Birmingham, for £65. She was renamed *Halmay III*.

Little is known of her until 1958, when she was docked at Bristol as a houseboat, owned by Mr Elliot, a New Zealander. In 1962 she was bought by J.E. Houghton, of Bristol, for £150 who moved her to Weymouth by train, where she continued to be used as a houseboat. The boat had been extensively altered and a superstructure had been added.

In 1987 she again changed hands, but soon afterwards sank at her moorings during a storm. By the end of the year she was lying derelict on the Fleet side of Chesil Beach and in September 1987 was due to be burned by a party of Royal Engineers helping with a beach clean up. However, fortunately, she was recognised as an old pulling lifeboat by the Weymouth's Honorary Secretary, Barney Morris, who positively identified her as *Ryder*. Berney then arranged with Lt Col Ron Overd, Commandant of the Royal Engineers camp at Wyke Regis and coincidentally a Looe man, for her recovery to Weymouth.

She was moved to the premises of Devonish Breweries at Brewers Quay in Weymouth, and they funded her restoration. She was restored to her original with the Brewery intending to place her on display in the 1990s. However, she was left outside in Weymouth, and gradually deteriorated.

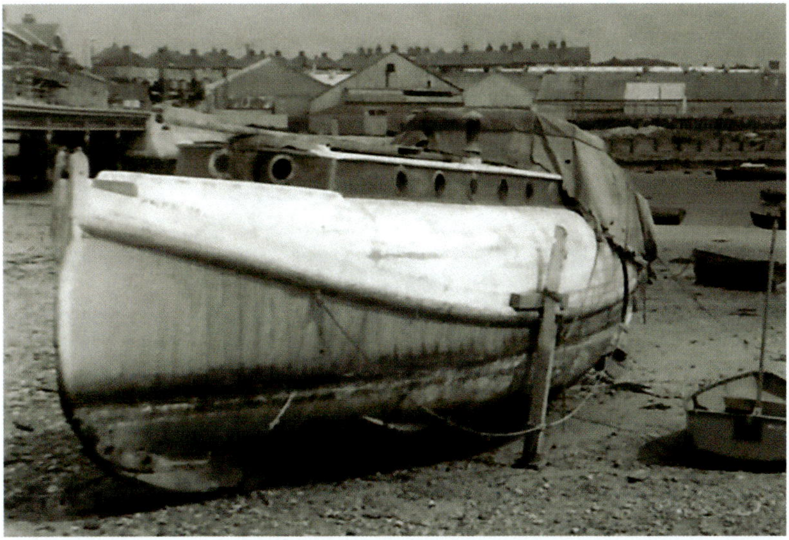

◀ Ryder after being converted into a houseboat with a superstructure covering her hull. (By courtesy of Looe RNLI)

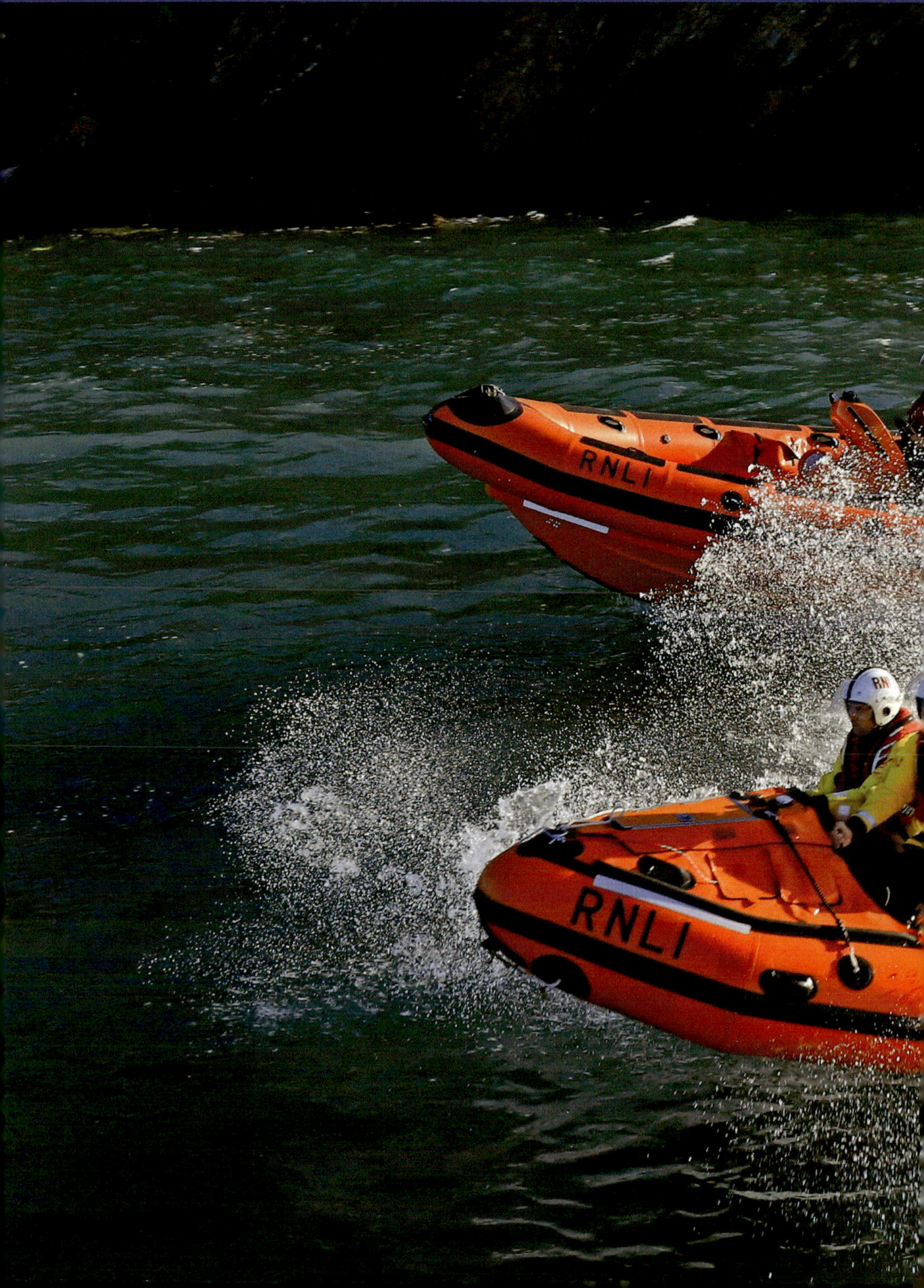
RNLI
RNLI

ONGUE II • D CLASS INFLATABLE D-741 OLLIE NAISMITH

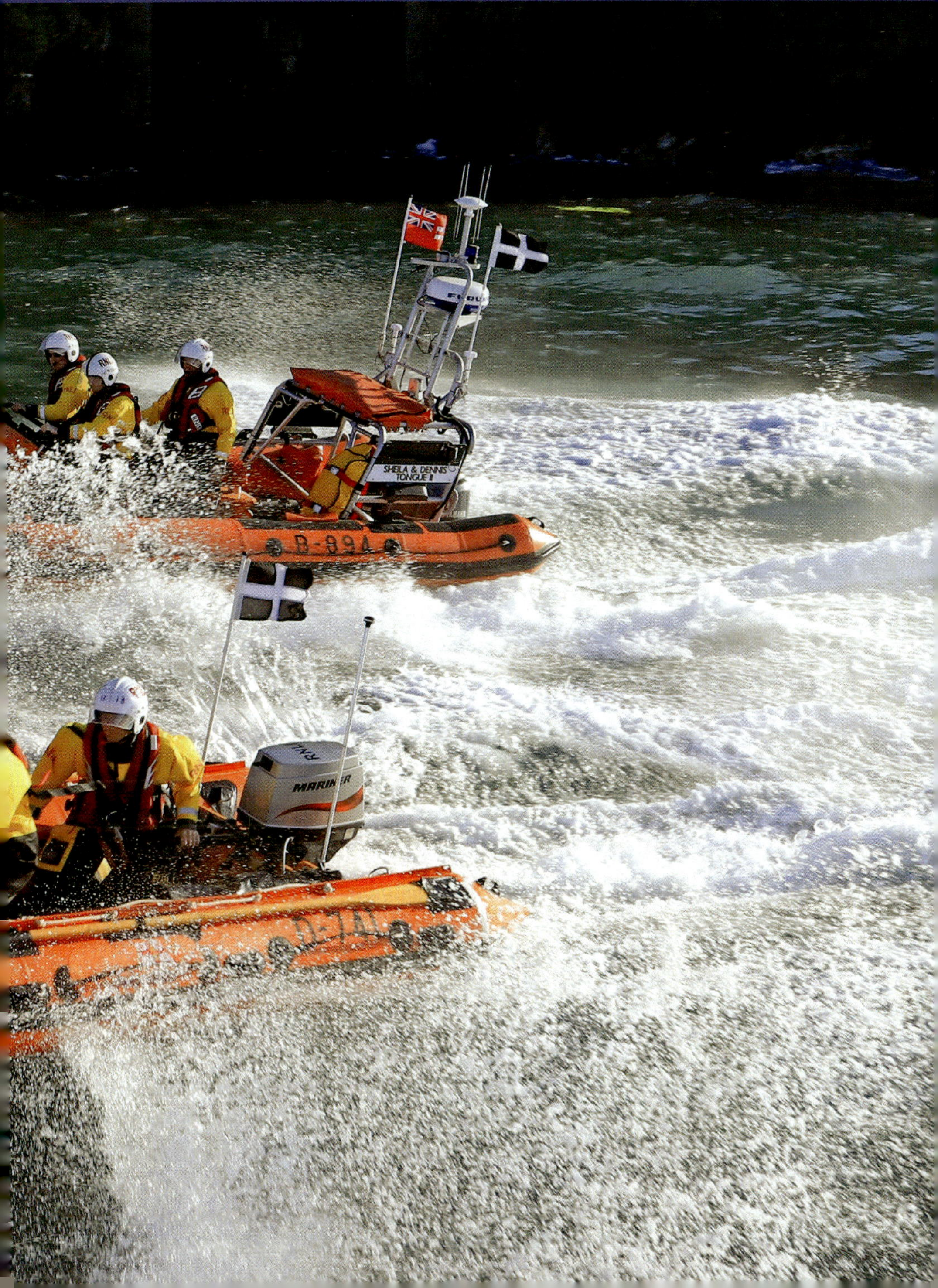

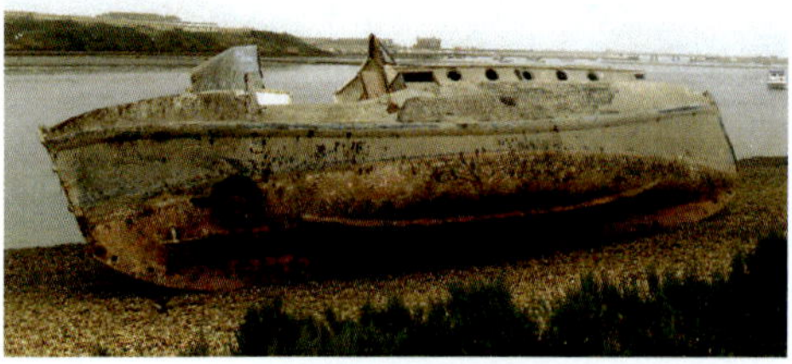

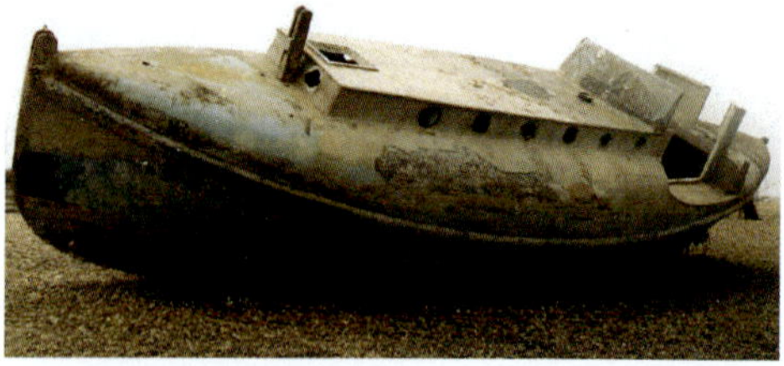

▲ Ryder was found derelict on Chesil Beach, Dorset after breaking from her moorings during a storm.

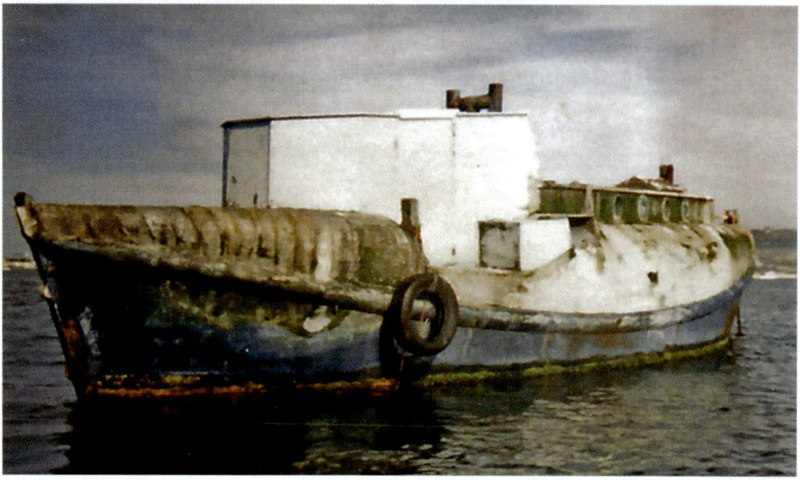

▶ Ryder in use as a houseboat. (Photos by courtesy of Looe RNLI)

In 1994 steps were taken to bring her back to Looe. However, this could not be achieved and in 1995 the Polperro Harbour Trustees stepped in and decided to recover and restore her to a seaworthy condition, and display her as a major exhibit at the Heritage Museum.

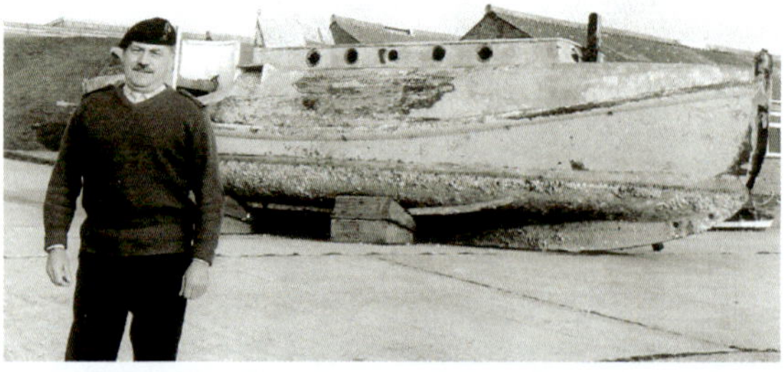

▼ Lt Col Ron Overd with the semi-derelict Ryder at the start of the process of saving her.

On 5 April 1995 she returned to Cornwall on a low-loader, and was placed at the quay of English China Clays, in Fowey, before being transferred onto the Bodinnick Ferry and shipped across the river to Alan Toms' boatyard at Polruan.

At Polruan *Ryder* was fully restored over the course of three years. The restoration was completed on 29 July 1998 and her launch was witnessed by about 150 people. *Ryder* was then taken to sea for trials under oars, crewed by members of the East Caradon Gig Club, and there followed a number of public displays of the former lifeboat around her native county.

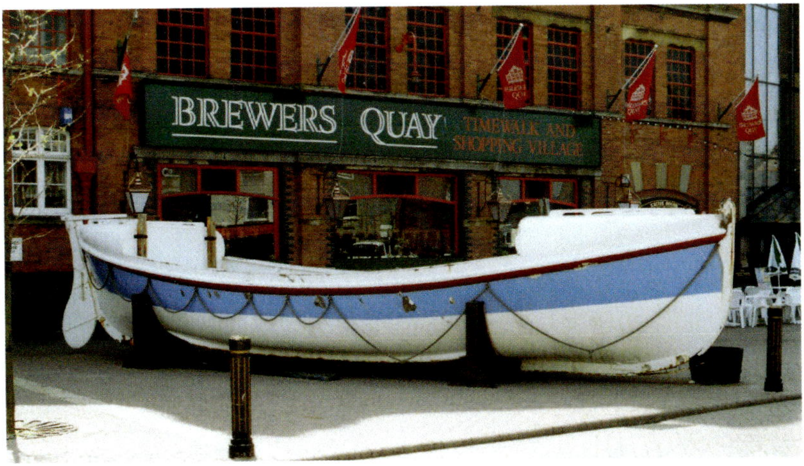

◀ Ryder outside Brewers Quay, Weymouth, having been restored to her original appearance. The late Alan Hilman was instrumental in saving Ryder.

On 1 August 1998 she was taken to Polperro harbour, being escorted in by Looe's D class inflatable *Spirit of the RAOC* and Fowey's 14m Trent *Maurice and Joyce Hardy*, which was in attendance for the event. She was berthed alongside the Heritage Museum and, after a short rededication by Dick Joliff a retired fisherman and local lay preacher, the inaugural celebrations were led by round-the-world yachtsman Tony Bullimore, who officially welcomed *Ryder* for public display.

On 2 August 1998 she was taken to Falmouth, where she participated in the display of 'Lifeboats Through the Ages'. She led the parade of old boats over to St Mawes, before she was rowed back. She was crewed by the Falmouth Gig Club and coxed by Toby West, a retired Falmouth Coxswain.

▼ Ryder off Falmouth in August 1998. The GPS on Falmouth's 17m Severn The Will measured her speed at a creditable 4.38 knots.

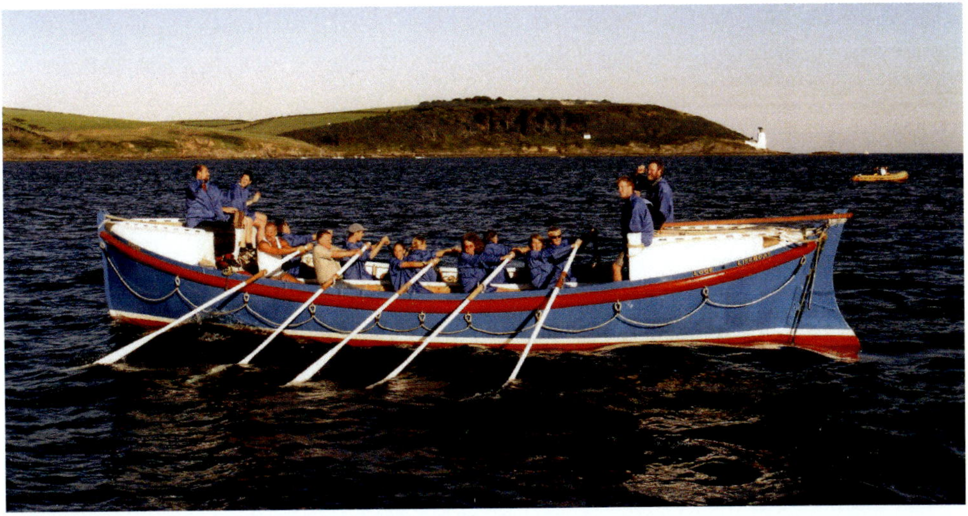

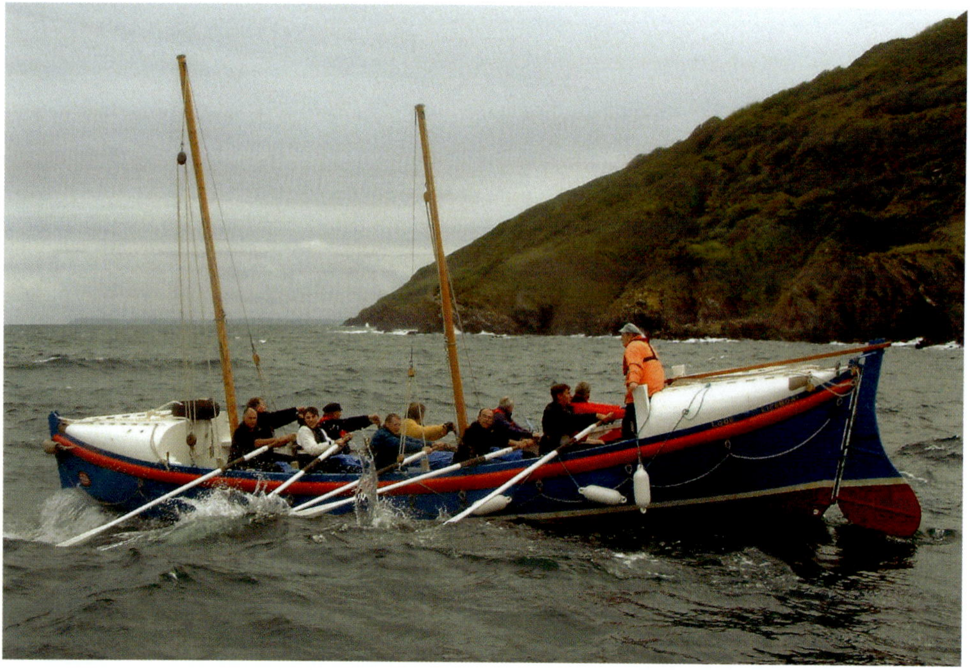

▲ Ryder with volunteers pulling at the oars off the Cornish coast, June 2002. The restoration project was dedicated to the bravery of the men who went out in her during her time at Looe. She has been displayed at the Heritage Museum in Polperro, where visitors can see her. (Paul Richards)

On 30 August 1998 *Ryder* returned to Looe, where she was escorted in by both the station's ILB and the local gig *Ryder*, which was named after the old lifeboat. She received a very enthusiastic welcome, particularly from relatives of former crew members.

Further developments took place in 1999. To help preserve *Ryder*, Project Ryder became a Registered Charity on 4 March. On 24 July Alfie Orchard and George Phillips, who were connected to Padstow lifeboat, visited the Museum. Alfie, aged 91, was crew from 1928 to 1930 in the station's second *Arab* lifeboat and was also bowman on Padstow's first motor lifeboat, *Princess Mary*. Both were taken out and then helped to row *Ryder* back to port.

On 27 August 1999 *Ryder* was taken to sea under sail for the first time. She handled better than was expected, in force three winds. She was light of her service weight by about five or six hundredweight, and needed a bit more ballast. At sea, she was found to be lively even in a force four, and Chairman Tony White said: "How her original crew ever kept a decent stroke in the dark, with a gale blowing I don't know. We have the utmost admiration for them!" As the boat has been taken to sea on a regular basis, her crew gradually acquired skill and gained insights into how the pulling boats were handled.

Ryder has been a regular attendee at the annual ex lifeboat gathering which takes place during

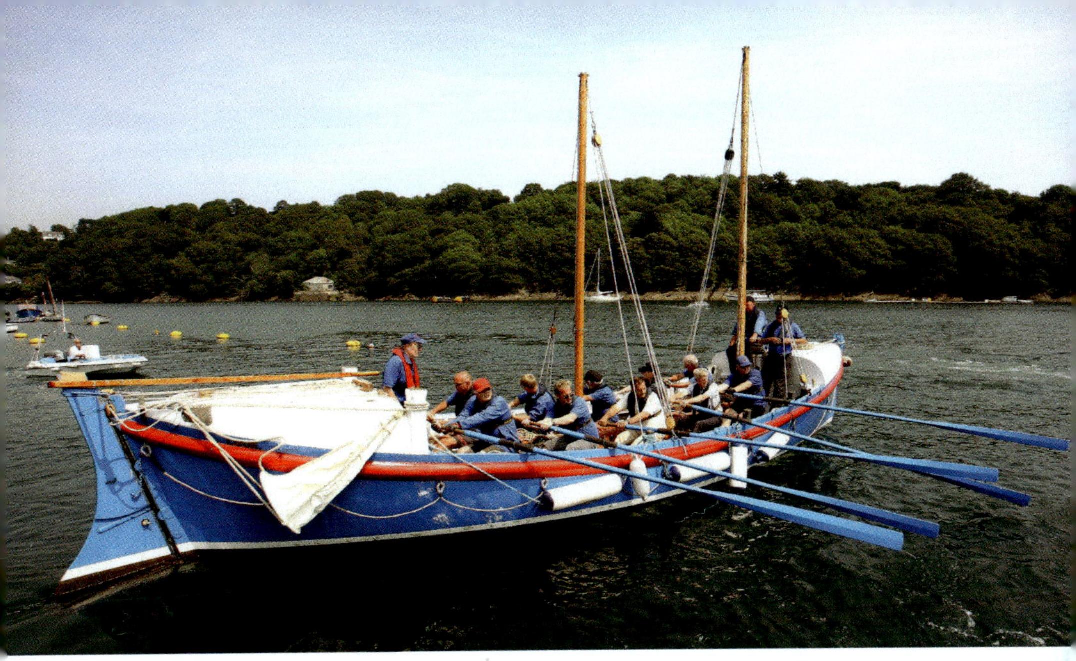

the summer at Fowey. Volunteers can row her round the estuary, pulling at the oars for an authentic lifeboat experience. In 2006 she was involved in a reconstruction of the rescue of the steamer *Suevic* by the Lizard lifeboat, which was the most lives to be saved in a single rescue, and on 21 September 2011 a Dart RNLI crew rowed *Ryder* in the Great London river race.

In May 2015 *Ryder* was taken further afield, being taken by road from Polruan to Courtmacsherry in Cork, Ireland to take part in the *Lusitania* Centenary event being, re-enacting the part played by Courtmacsherry lifeboat *Kezia Gwilt*.

▲ Ryder taking part in the ex lifeboat gathering at Fowey, July 2006. (Nicholas Leach)

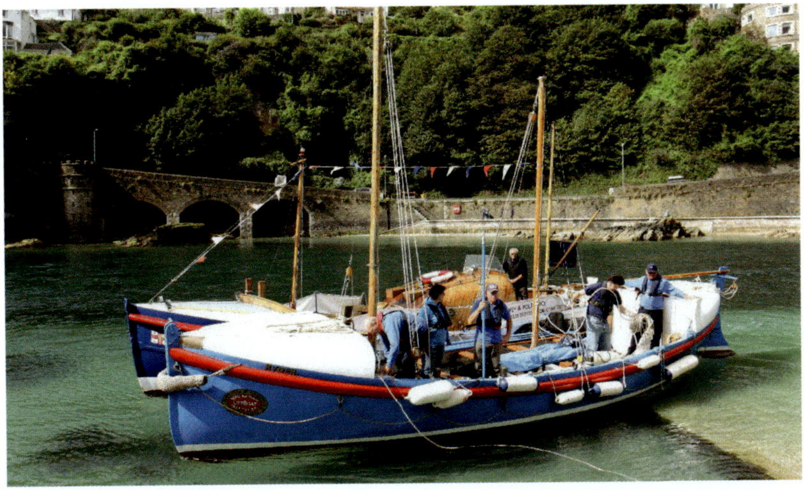

◀ Ryder in Looe alongside William Cantrell Ashley, another old lifeboat, for the naming ceremony of the new D class inflatable Ollie Naismith (D-741), July 2011. (Nicholas Leach)

1991 – A NEW INSHORE LIFEBOAT STATION

In 1991, following a review of life-saving cover at Looe and the surrounding coastline, the RNLI resolved that, subject to the provision of suitable shore facilities, a summer only D class inshore lifeboat would be allocated for one season's operational evaluation. A relief ILB, D-355, was sent to the station and remained until the summer of 1994, by when the station had proved its worth. Shore facilities and accommodation for the ILB were found in an existing building, generously provided by East Looe Town Trust, at the head of the beach at East Looe, close to the old lifeboat house.

During 1992 several services were carried out, with the first, on 19 June, seeing the ILB and her volunteer crew saving a yacht and her two crew. On 29 July a seven people were landed from a cabin

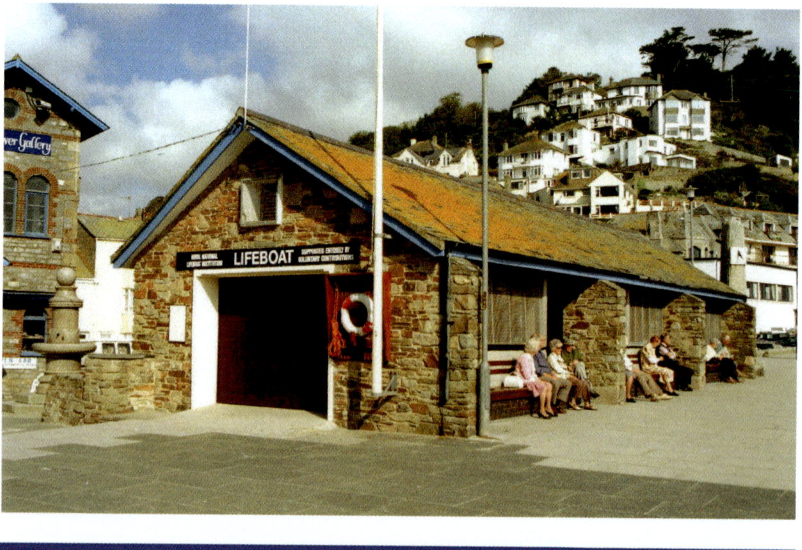

▶ The first boathouse used for the inshore lifeboat was situated at East Looe, close to the beach and adjacent to the old lifebot house, pictured in October 1997. (Nicholas Leach)

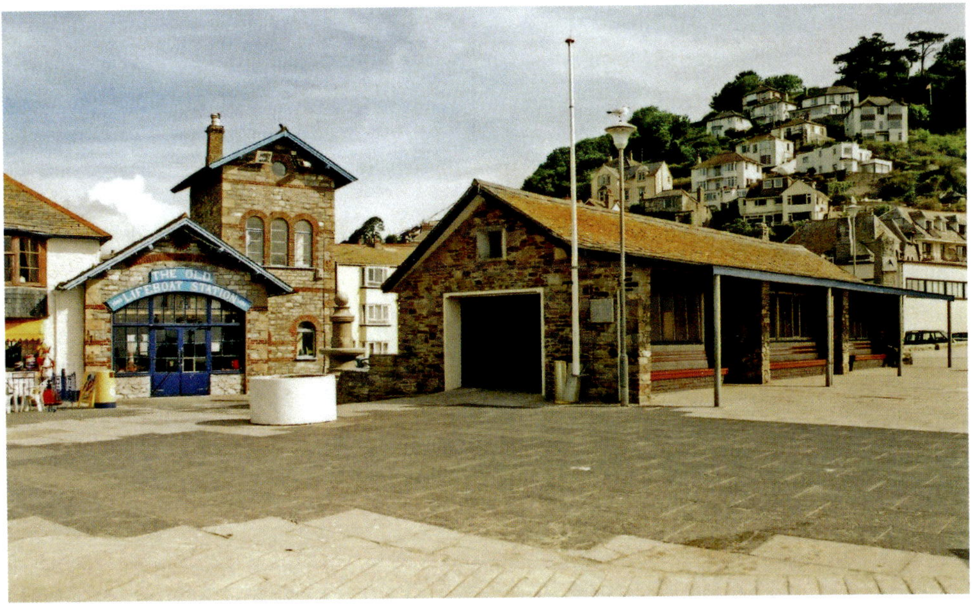

▲ The first building used as a boathouse for the inshore lifeboat, located adjacent to the original lifeboat house, pictured in October 1997. (Nicholas Leach)

cruiser which got into difficulty, and later the same day four people were saved after they got cut off by the tide. During September 1992 three fishing vessels were assisted, and the value of the newly-established ILB station was clear.

In 1994 the relief D class inflatable D-396 *Starting Point*, which had been built in 1989 and funded by Frizzell Insurance and Blakesley village, was on station until 12 August 1994, when the new ILB *Spirit of the RAOC* (D-461) took up station. The station's first newly-built ILB was funded by 12 Supply Regiment, the Royal Logistic Corps, and was in action three days after she arrived, launching to help a broken down motor boat.

The original ILB accommodation proved to be unsuitable in the long term and so, in 1998, the ILB was moved to a new boathouse at Middleton's Corner on East Looe Quay. The building was acquired in 1997 and converted to house the ILB and provide crew facilities, while a davit was installed on the adjacent quayside to launch the ILB into the river. The new building was formally opened on 11 July 1998 by Lt Cdr Brian Miles, the RNLI's Director, following a service of dedication led by the Rev Robert Hilton and the Rev Brian McQuillen.

By this time the ILBs and their crews were being called on with increasing frequency. In 1997 almost twenty services had been performed and a dozen effective rescues were undertaken the following year. The range of causalities was considerable, and included people stranded on cliffs, a youth fallen from the bridge crossing the river, children cut by the tide, and swimmers, as well as dinghies, inflatables and dive support craft. Up to 2001, representing a decade of operations, the various D class ILBs launched 190 times and saved forty-four lives.

A new lifeboat station

In September 2001 a site on the sea front was acquired by the RNLI from the East Looe Town Trust for a new lifeboat house, and in January 2002 a package of improvements, costing approximately £1.5 million, was announced, including plans for a new lifeboat station, subject to planning permission, with provision for a second, larger ILB. The scheme envisaged the provision of a new Atlantic twin-engined rigid-inflatable which would require a new lifeboat station to be built. The Albatross crazy golf site on East Looe Quay, about 100 yards nearer the sea than Middleton's Corner, was identified as the best location.

In 2002 the RNLI Trustees agreed that an Atlantic 75 inshore lifeboat would be co-located with the D class ILB at Looe, and construction of the new lifeboat station commenced in the autumn of that year. The second, larger lifeboat had greater capabilities than the D class inflatable, which had been tested to the limit on service during the previous decade. The Atlantic would greatly enhance the crew's abilities to respond to more demanding situations that had faced them in the D class ILB, and improve rescue coverage around the coast off Looe, and out to sea.

As well as housing two ILBs, the new building, built out of stone and slate, provided modern facilities for the crew and also had space for an RNLI souvenir shop, which went on to become very busy, particularly

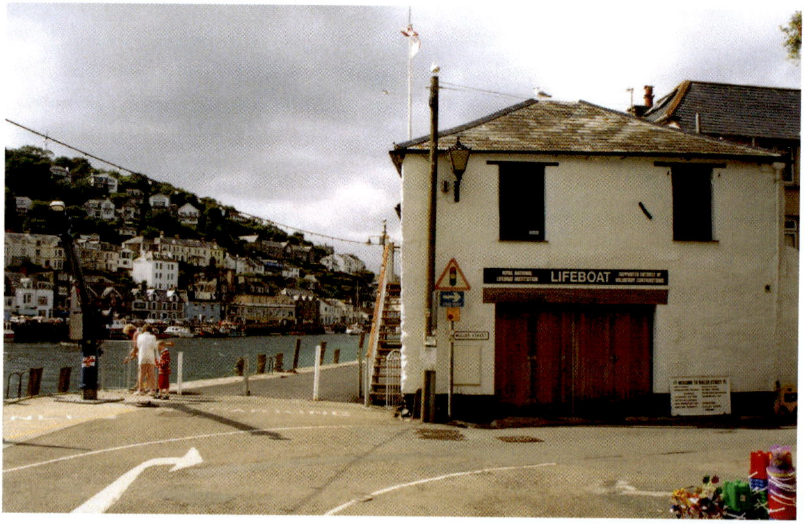

▶ The building at Middleton's Corner that was converted for the ILB, with the launching for on the right. (Nicholas Leach)

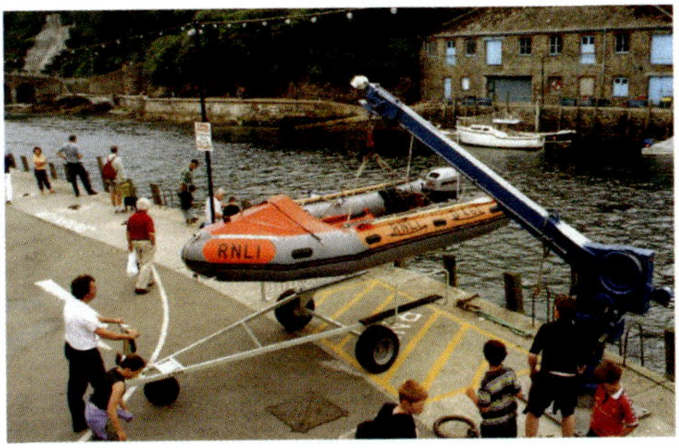

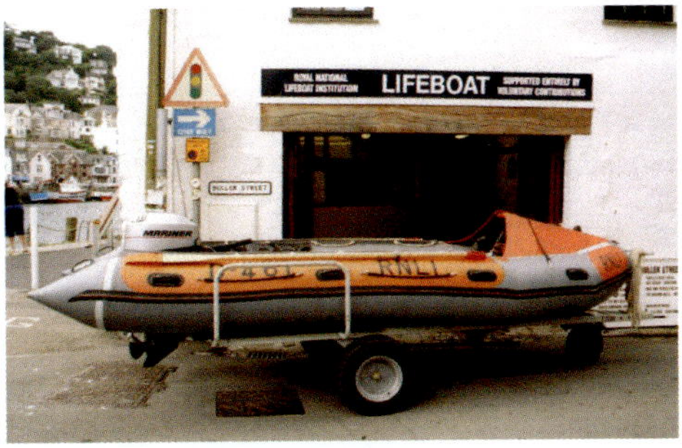

▲ Spirit of the RAOC (D-461) on her trailer outside the ILB house at Middleton's Corner, July 2001. (Nicholas Leach)

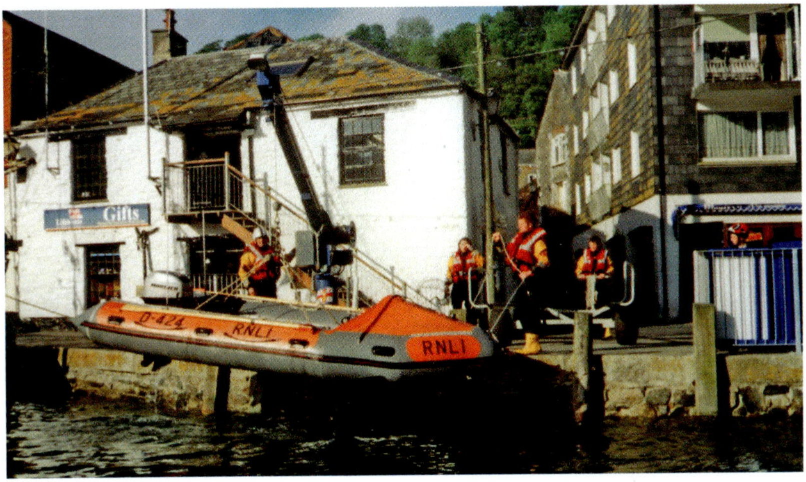

◀ Relief D class D-424 City of Chester being lowered into the water off East Looe Quay. (RNLI)

during the summer months. The first floor had a large training room, office facilities and an observation point from which the safety of the ILBs could be monitored. Changing facilities on the ground floor were adjacent to the boathall, where both ILBs and their respective launch vehicles were kept. Building work started on 25 November 2002, and the keys were handed over to the RNLI on 2 October 2003.

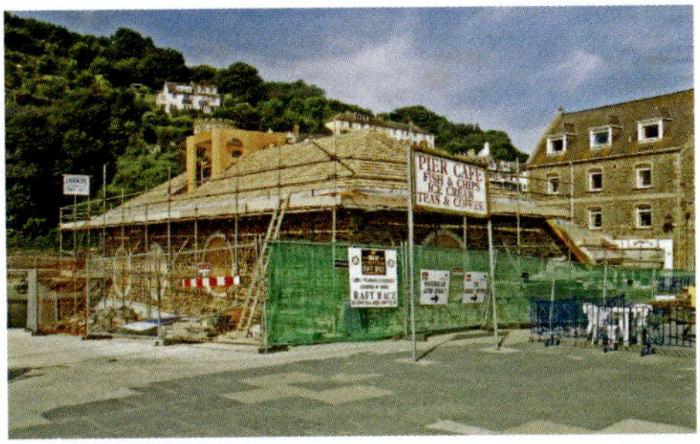

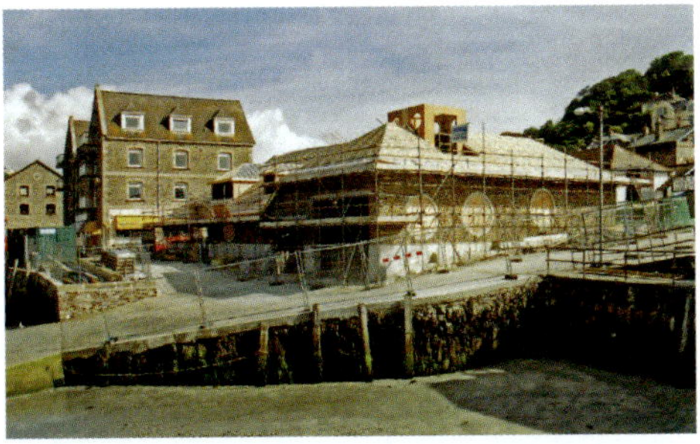

▲ The lifeboat house under construction at East Looe in June 2003. As part of the project, the RNLI, in conjunction with Looe Harbour Commissioners, rebuilt the boat slipway into the river. (Nicholas Leach)

▶ The lifeboat house at East Looe, with a slipway into the river, built in 2002-03 for Atlantic and D class ILBs, pictured in March 2015. (Nicholas Leach)

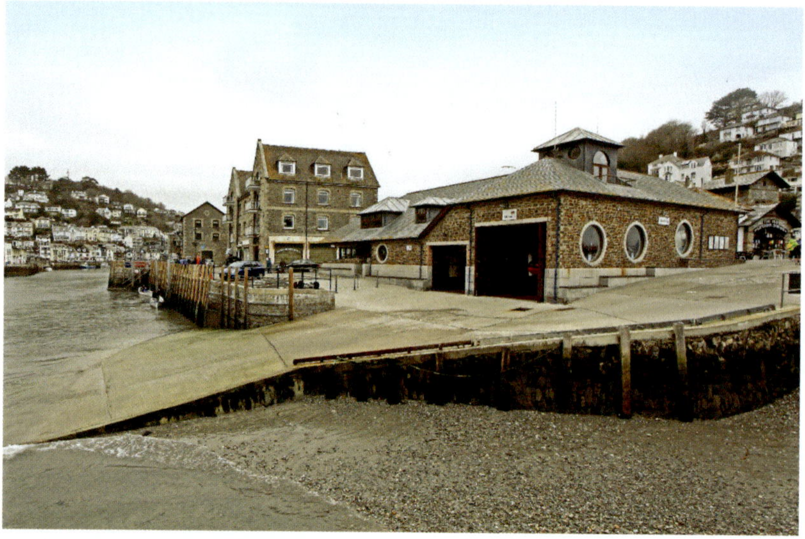

Before the new boathouse had been completed, a new D class inflatable arrived to replace *Spirit of the RAOC* (D-461), which has been at the station for eight years. The arrival of the new boat in March 2002 was the first stage in the renewal and upgrading of the station. The new ILB, named *Regina Mary* (D-574), was formally placed on station at 6pm on 5 March 2002. She was named and dedicated on 22 June 2002 during the port's three-day festival of the sea, an event held every two years and which has a strong RNLI flavour.

▼ The scene during the naming of Regina Mary (D-574) at Middleton's Corner, 22 June 2002. (Paul Richards)

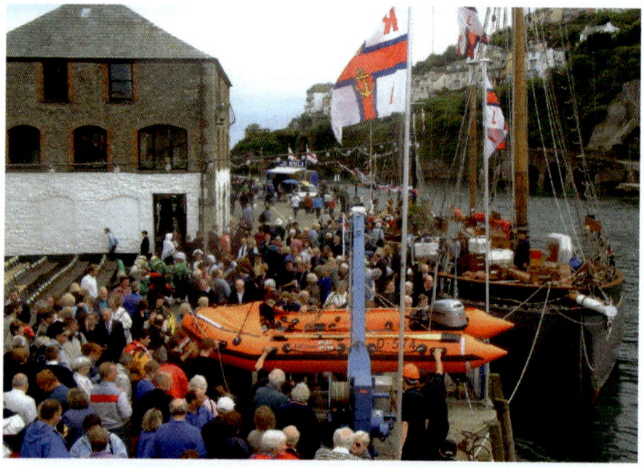

For the naming ceremony, the all-weather Trent class lifeboat from Fowey, *Maurice and Joyce Hardy,* was in attendance. The event was held outside the lifeboat house at Middleton's Corner, with a large number of guests and festival visitors occupying the quayside area. Present at the ceremony was Lawrence Allan, from Somerset, a governor of the RNLI, who had given the money for the lifeboat in 1996. Regina Mary Lewis, after whom the lifeboat was named, performed the christening ceremony, pouring champagne over the ILB's bow, after which the boat was lowered into the water, via the quayside davit, for a demonstration.

The day before the naming ceremony, the Earl and Countess of Wessex had visited the station,

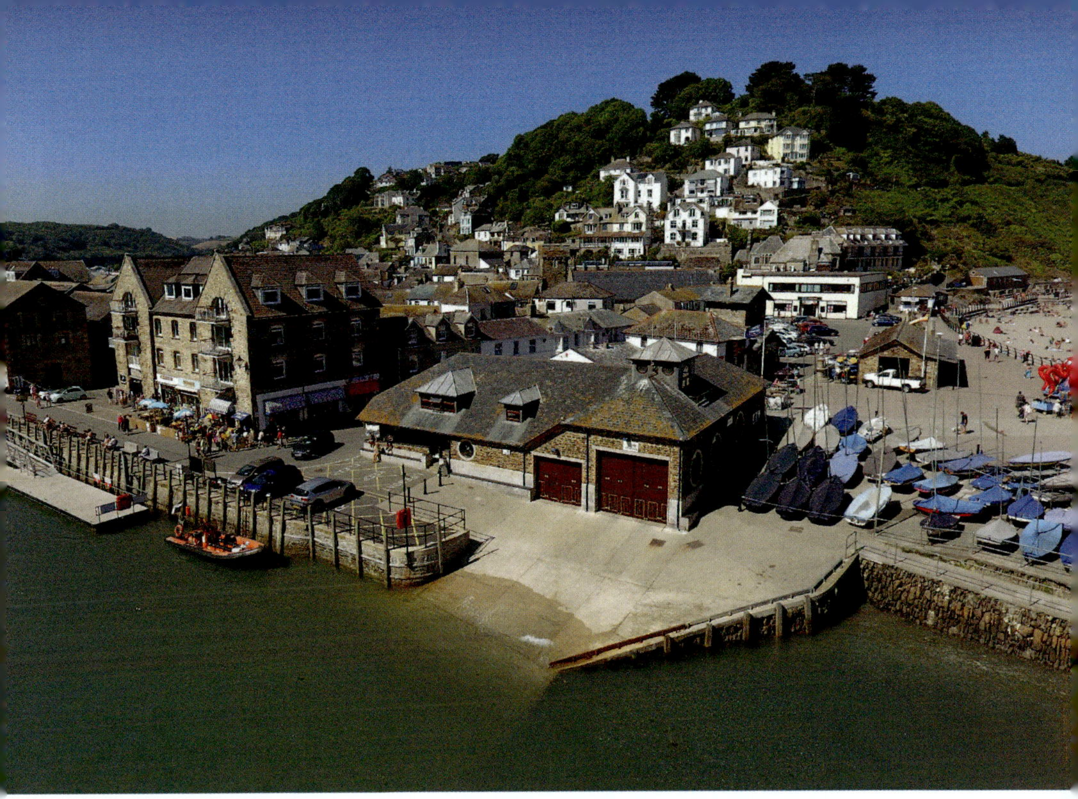

while on the Sunday after the ceremony a service of rededication was held for the restored lifeboat *Ryder*, which served at Looe from 1902 until 1930 (see chapter 2). It was also stated that, during the first ten years of ILB operations at Looe, between 1992 and 2002, the ILBs had launched 238 times, rescued 187 people and saved 55 lives.

▲ The lifeboat house at East Looe. (EFAS)

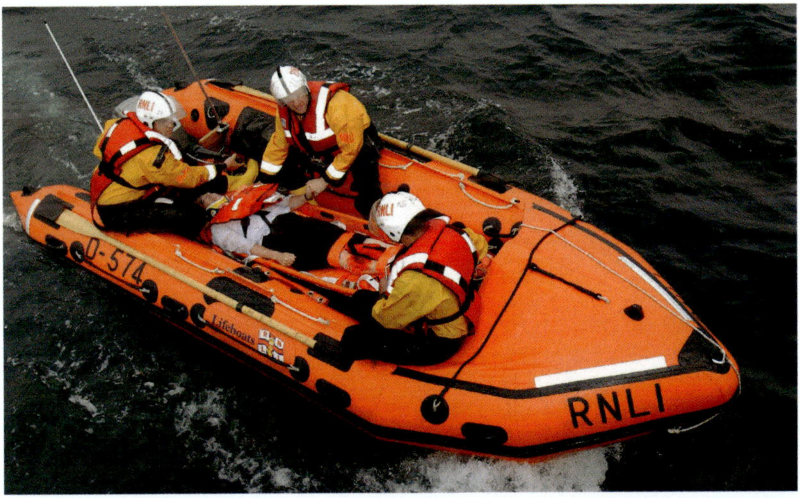

◀ Regina Mary (D-574) on exercise on 18 July 2005, when the RNLI launched its 'Train One, Save Many' campaign. (By courtesy of the RNLI)

▶ Relief Atlantic 75 B-700 Susan Peacock (top) during crew training in 2003 prior to an Atlantic going on station; and the station's own Atlantic 75 Alan and Margaret (B-793) arriving by road at Looe for the first time, October 2003 (middle). (Ian Foster)

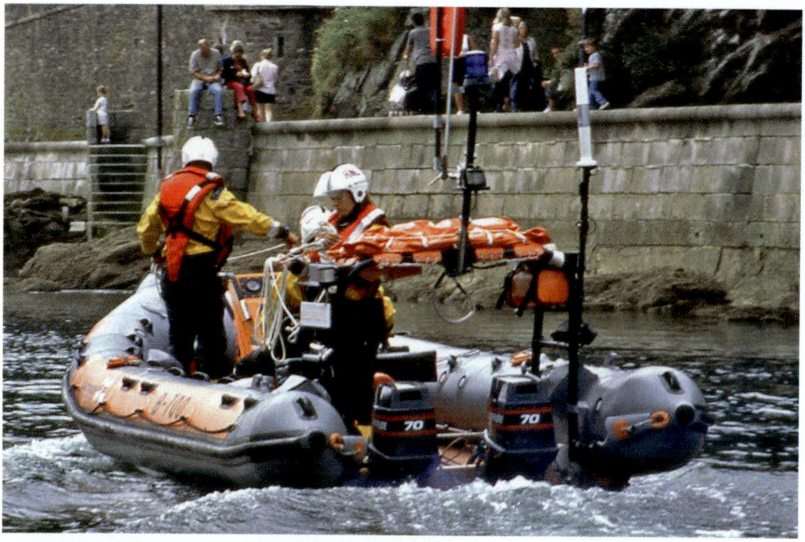

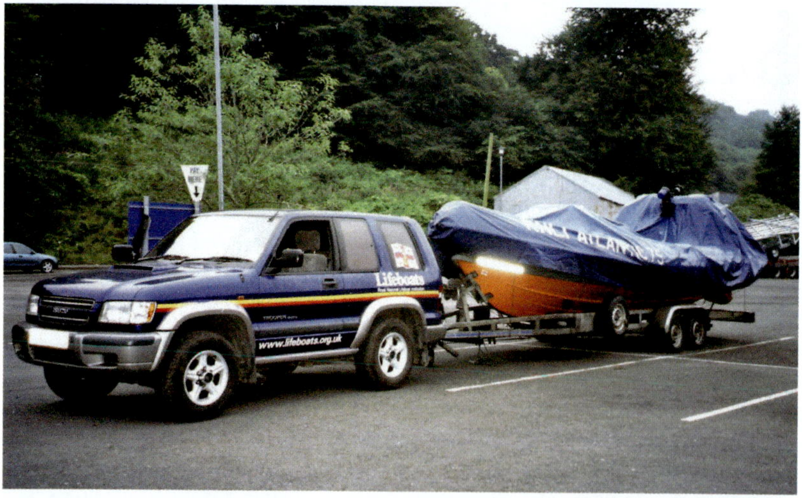

▼ Fowey and Plymouth lifeboats in attendance at Looe for the naming of Atlantic 75 Alan and Margaret (B-793), 18 October 2003. (Paul Richards)

▼ (right) Ryder on hand for the naming of Alan and Margaret (B-793). (Paul Richards)

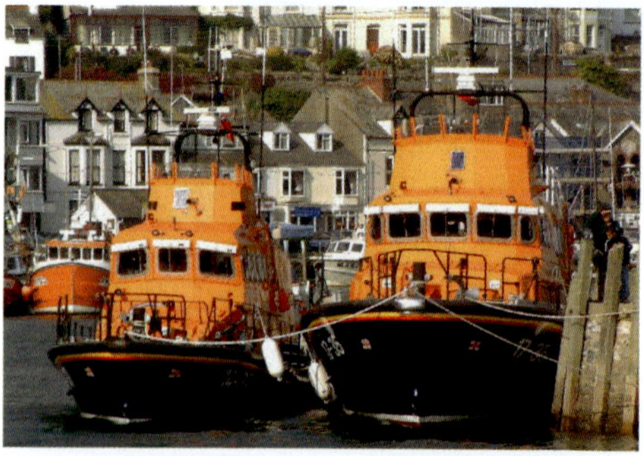

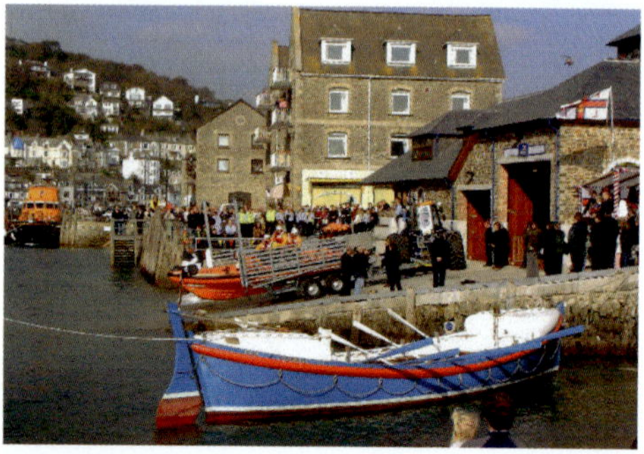

With the new boathouse nearing completion, crew training and familiarisation on an Atlantic 75 was needed, and on 6 August 2003 the relief Atlantic *Susan Peacock* (B-700) arrived at the station. She was the first Atlantic 75 to be built and had been used in the RNLI's Relief Fleet as well as for training at a number of stations. The boat was kept ashore on a trailer, from which she was launched so that the crew could undertake training.

Within hours of her arrival, B-700 was called out to assist with a rescue as the crew were already at sea learning about the equipment on and capabilities of the new craft. Three youngsters were in difficulty on a large rubber ring, so *Regina Mary* (D-574) was launched, and the youngsters were safely returned to shore. The crew of the Atlantic, as they headed back to station, assisted two children on a surf board.

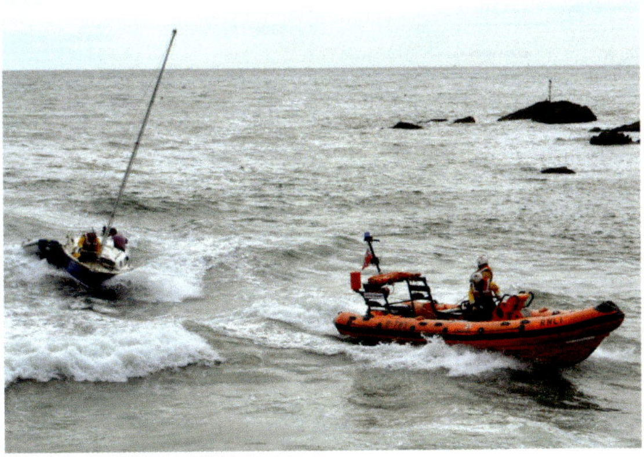

▲ Atlantic 75 *Alan and Margaret* (B-793) towing a small yacht to safety. (RNLI)

During the rest of August and into September crew training continued on the Atlantic with an intensive schedule, while the finishing touches were made to the new lifeboat house. By the end of September the new building was ready, and the Atlantic was moved inside. A drive-on drive-off launching trolley was supplied, and this was hauled into position by a Talus MB-4H tractor. This fully marinised vehicle could take the

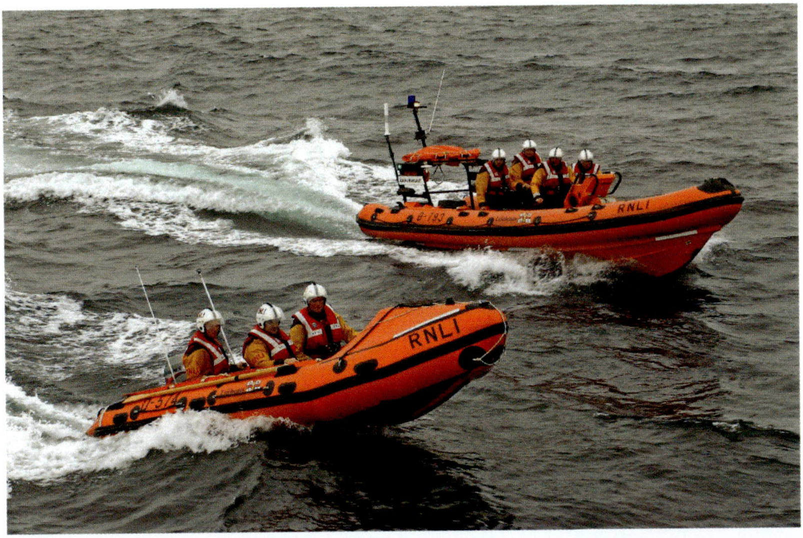

◀ Atlantic 75 *Alan and Margaret* (B-793) and *Regina Mary* (D-574) on exercise off Looe, June 2005. (Nicholas Leach)

▶ The naming ceremony of Ollie Naismith (D-741), 9 July 2011. Support for the appeal to fund the ILB was overwhelming from the local community and in just eight months more than £84,000 had been raised. (Nicholas Leach)

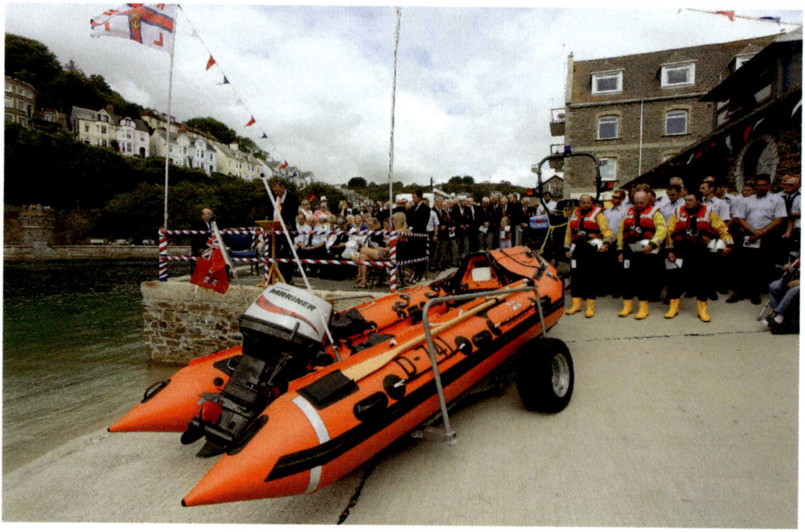

boat on its carriage out of the river at low tide and into the sea and surf.

In late September 2003 the station's own new Atlantic 75, *Alan and Margaret* (B-793), arrived and on 2 October 2003 was declared operational, thus completing the upgrading of the station. The new Atlantic was funded from the gift of Miss Elizabeth Beaton, and was named after the donor's parents by Miss Beaton during a ceremony on 18 October 2003. The donor and her mother decided to fund the lifeboat with money from her parents' estate. Alan Beaton, who lived in Earlswood Close, Bedgrove, with his wife Margaret, died aged 81 after a heart attack in October 1996. When Elizabeth realised she

▶ Tori Naismith pours the champagne over the bows of the new inshore lifeboat, naming Ollie Naismith (D-741) at the end of the ceremony, 9 July 2011. (Nicholas Leach)

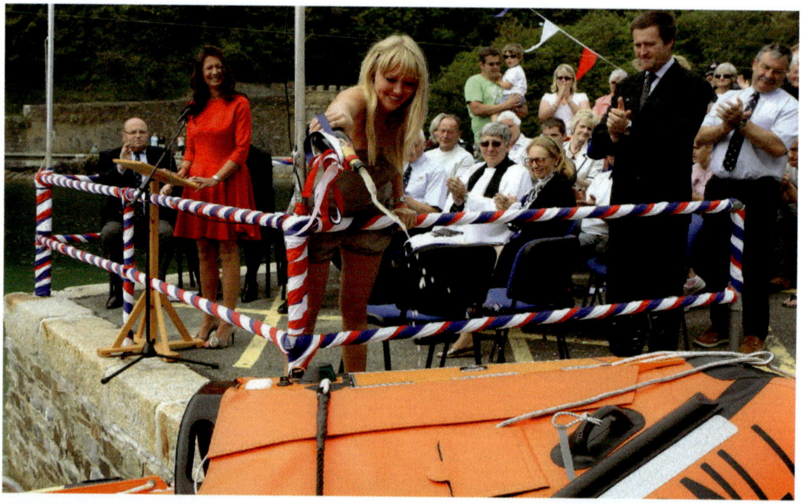

and her mother would have to pay inheritance tax if the money was not given to charity, they decided to buy the £81,600 boat outright.

At the ceremony, after the lifeboat had been named, the new lifeboat house was also formally opened by Lady Mary Holbarrow, JP, Lord Lieutenant of Cornwall, with the lifeboat then launching for a short demonstration afloat.

The volunteer crew, operating from a state-of-the-art purpose-built boathouse, now had two new lifeboats, as the new century got under way, and were in a position to respond faster and more effectively to incidents. Every year, the volunteer crew are called out to a wide variety of incidents, and throughout the 2000s averaged about twenty-five call-outs a year.

An unusual shout took place on Wednesday 3 June 2009 when the lifeboat crew put out in the early

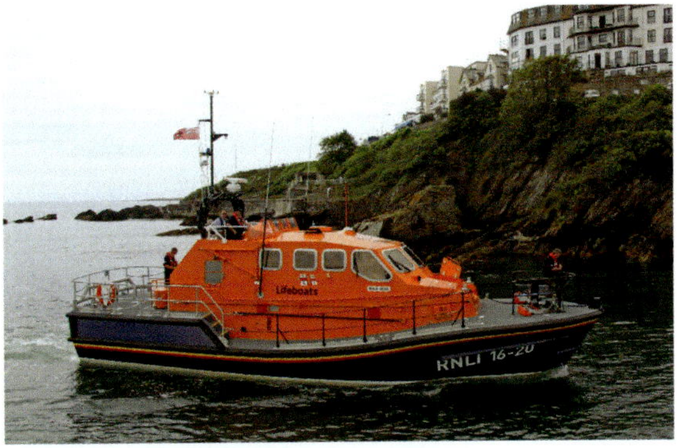

◀ Lizard's new 16m Tamar lifeboat Rose arriving at Looe for the naming of the new D class inflatable Ollie Naismith (D-741), 9 July 2011.

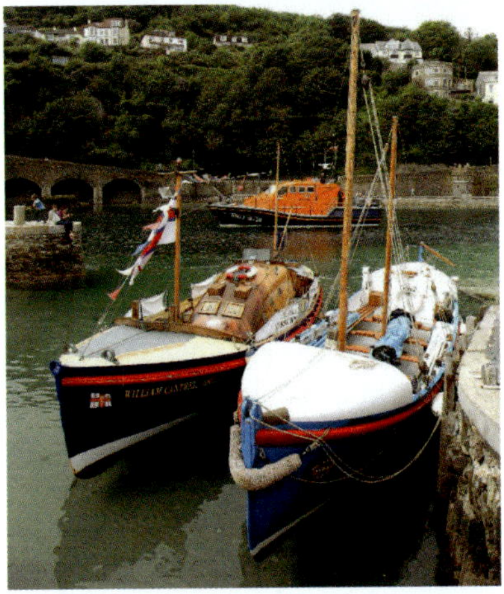

◀ Former lifeboats William Cantrell Ashley (on left) and Ryder at Looe for the naming of D-741.

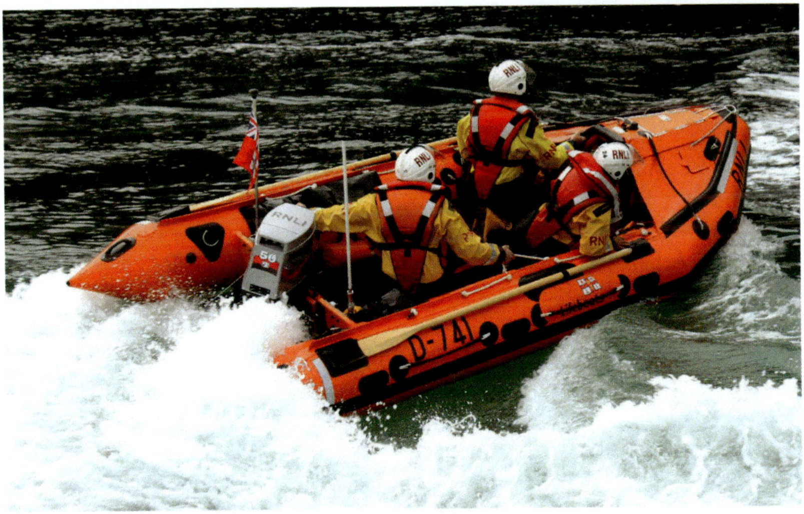

◀ The new D class inflatable Ollie Naismith (D-741) at the end of her naming ceremony, with her crew demonstrating the boat's capabilities, 9 July 2011. (Nicholas Leach)

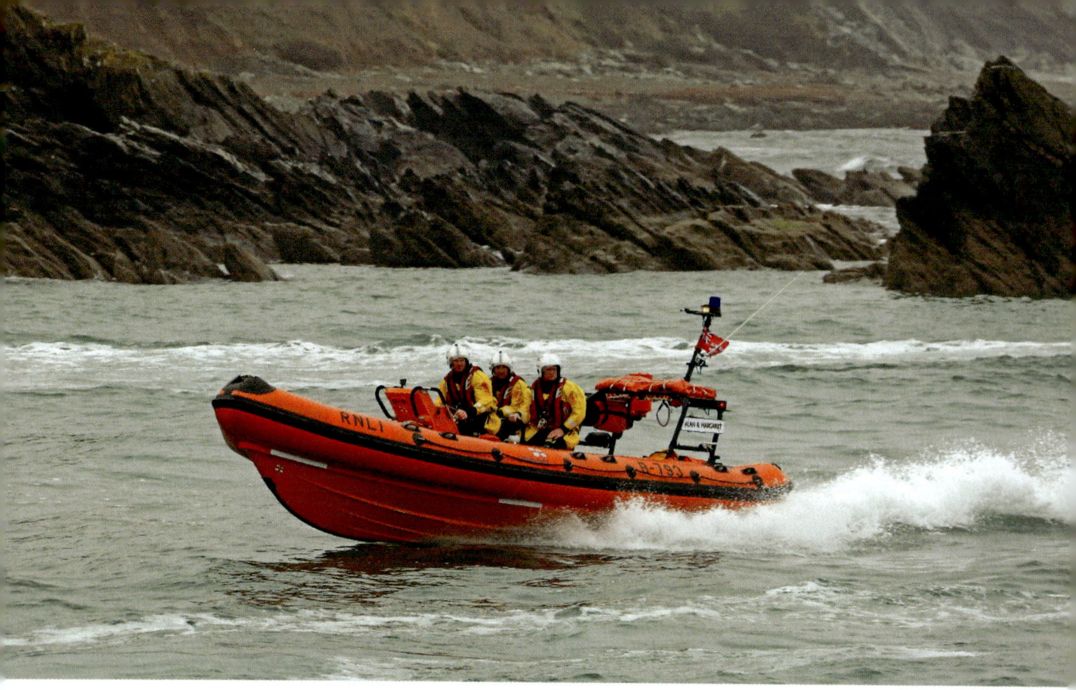

▲ Atlantic 75 Alan and Margaret (B-793) on exercise off Looe, May 2015. During her thirteen years of service at Looe (2003-2016), she was launched 252 times, rescued 208 people, and saved two lives. (Nicholas Leach)

afternoon to the aid of a couple after a swarm of bees had invaded their yacht a mile off the coast at Polperro. The bees forced the couple out of the steering cockpit onto the vessel's bow, while the crew, keeping safe in their drysuits and helmets, used smoke flares and water jets to disperse the bees.

Two new lifeboats

Towards the end of the decade, the station was allocated a new D class inshore lifeboat. A campaign to fund the boat in memory of Ollie Naismith, a local teenager who tragically died, aged nineteen, in a road traffic accident in 2009, was started. Following Ollie's death, his parents, Maxine and John Naismith, spearheaded the fund-raising and the appeal soon raised £84,000, more than double the original target, in just eight months and the new ILB, named *Ollie Naismith*, arrived at her station in November 2010.

The new boat, D-741, was named and dedicated at a ceremony heavy with emotion held at the lifeboat station on 9 July 2011, with hundreds of people in attendance. The service of dedication was led by the Reverend Brian McQuillen, who came to Looe specially for the service having retired earlier in the year. The ILB was handed into the care of the RNLI by John Naismith and was named by Ollie's mother, Maxine, and his sister, Tori. Speeches by the family recalled Ollie and his short life, with many of those present being overcome with emotion.

Lifeboat Operations Manager David Haines said: 'On behalf of Looe RNLI, it gives me great pleasure to accept the *Ollie Naismith* into our care. We're delighted with this new inshore lifeboat, which arrived on station in November. Since then, she has launched eleven times and assisted sixteen people. When the appeal was launched in March last year for £31,000, we never imagined we would be standing here today, with more than £84,000 raised.' It had been an outstanding effort by all those involved, and reflected the esteem in which Ollie was held.

Lizard's new 16m Tamar class lifeboat *Rose*, which was on passage to her station from the RNLI College in Poole, called in for the ceremony. The historic *Ryder* was also moored close to the ceremony site, along with *William Cantrell Ashley*, another old lifeboat then based in Looe. After the ceremony, *Rose* and her

▼ Lifeboat crew on hand to welcome HRH Duke and Duchess of Cornwall during their visit to Looe on 14 July 2014. (Simon Culliford, by courtesy of Looe RNLI)

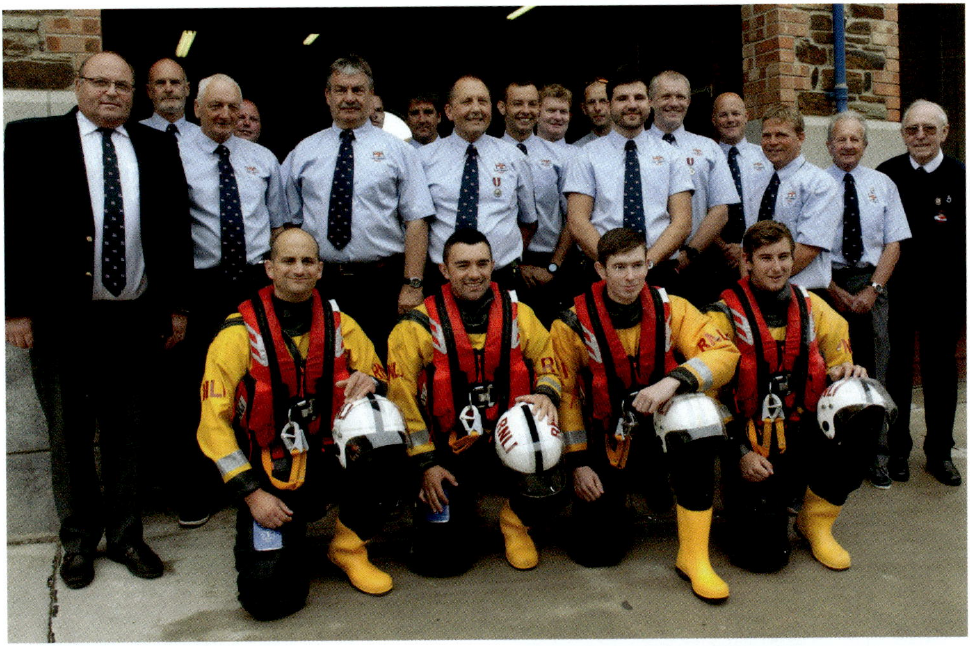

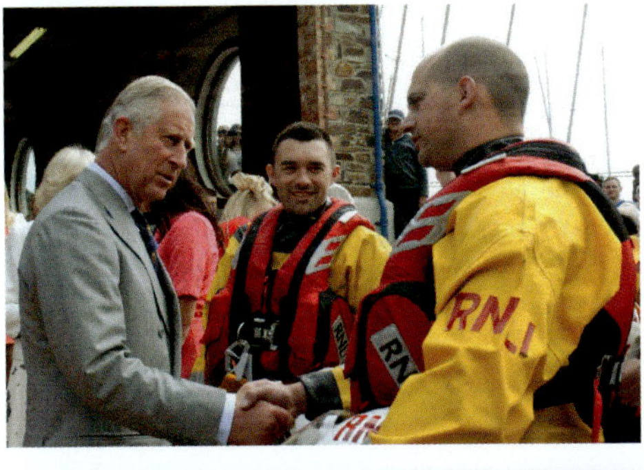

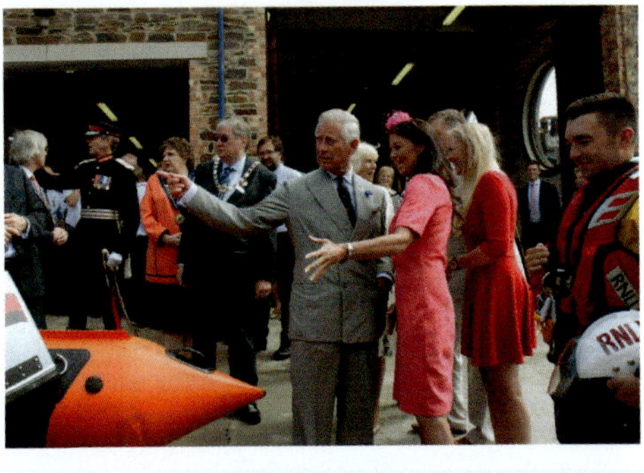

crew departed for the next leg of their training passage.

In July 2014 Prince Charles and Camilla, Duchess of Cornwall, visited Looe during their annual visit to the county. The Duke and Duchess wanted to meet people who had been affected by flooding and damage in the winter storms, as well as the men and women of the local emergency services. Thousands of people lined the river as the royal couple were driven through the town to the quay and the lifeboat house. They met crew and lifeboat volunteers, and talked to David Haines. The royal couple also spent some time with John and Maxine Naismith, and their daughter Tori.

By this time, a new Atlantic 85 for Looe had been scheduled into the RNLI's building programme. One of the last services undertaken by Atlantic 75 *Alan and Margaret* (B-793) came on 28 May 2016, when she joined lifeboats from

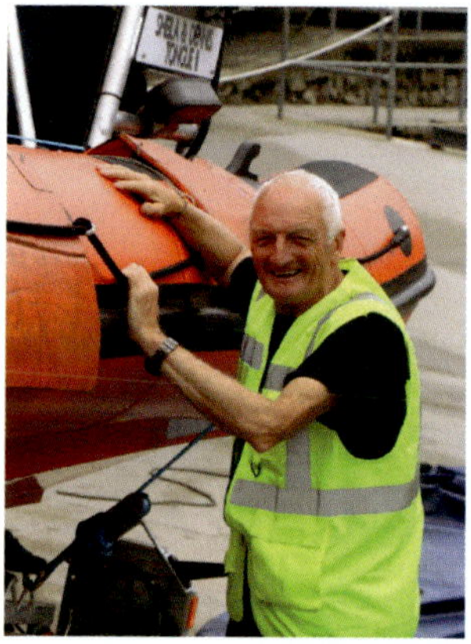

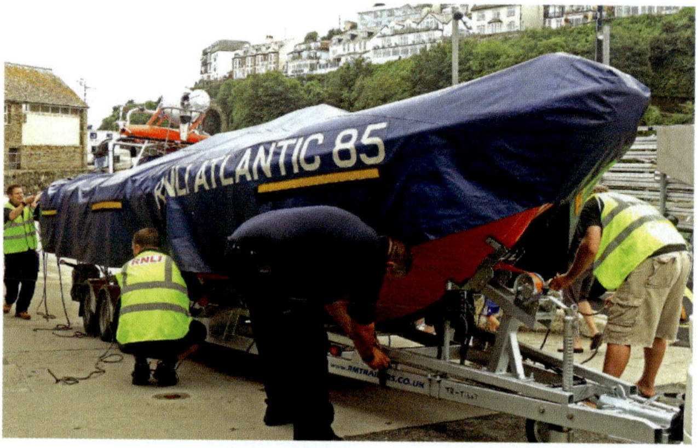

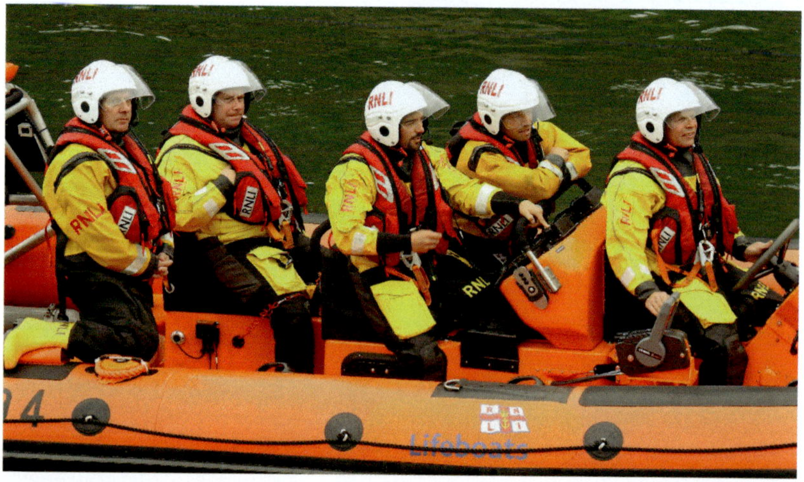

▲ The new Atlantic 85 *Sheila & Dennis Tongue II* (B-894) arrives on station, 5 September 2016, with Lifeboat Operations Manager David Haines (left) helping to get the boat ready. (Ian Foster)

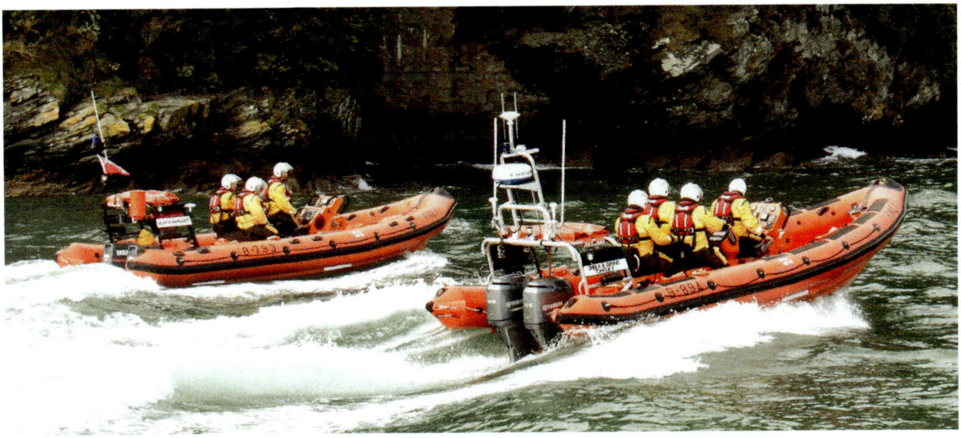

▲ The new Atlantic 85 Sheila & Dennis Tongue II (B-894) with her predecessor, Alan and Margaret (B-793), on 7 September 2016, just before the 85 took up operational duties. (Ian Foster)

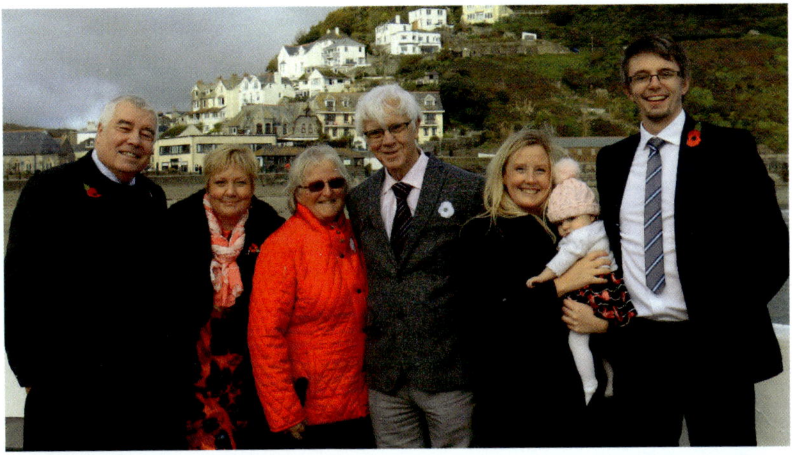

◀ The Tongue family in attendance at the naming ceremony. (Ian Foster)

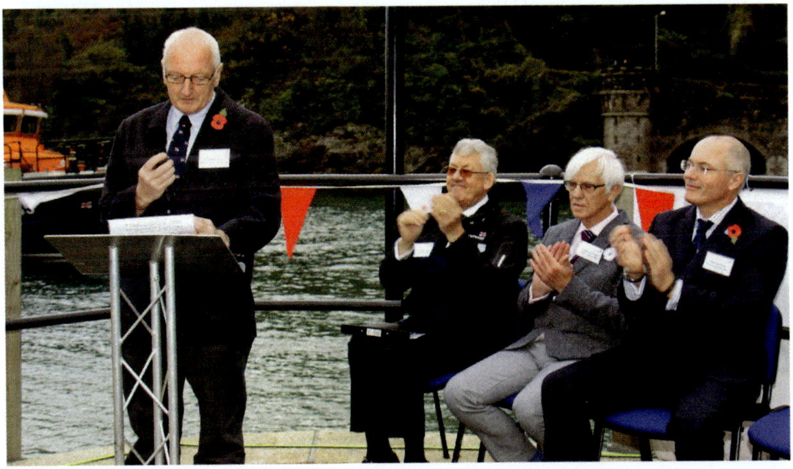

◀ Lifeboat Operations Manager David Haines speaking during the naming ceremony of the Atlantic 85 Sheila & Dennis Tongue II (B-894) on 12 November 2016. (Ian Foster)

▶ Plymouth lifeboat Sybil Mullen Glover in attendance at the naming for Atlantic 85 Sheila & Dennis Tongue II (B-894), 12 November 2016. (Ian Foster)

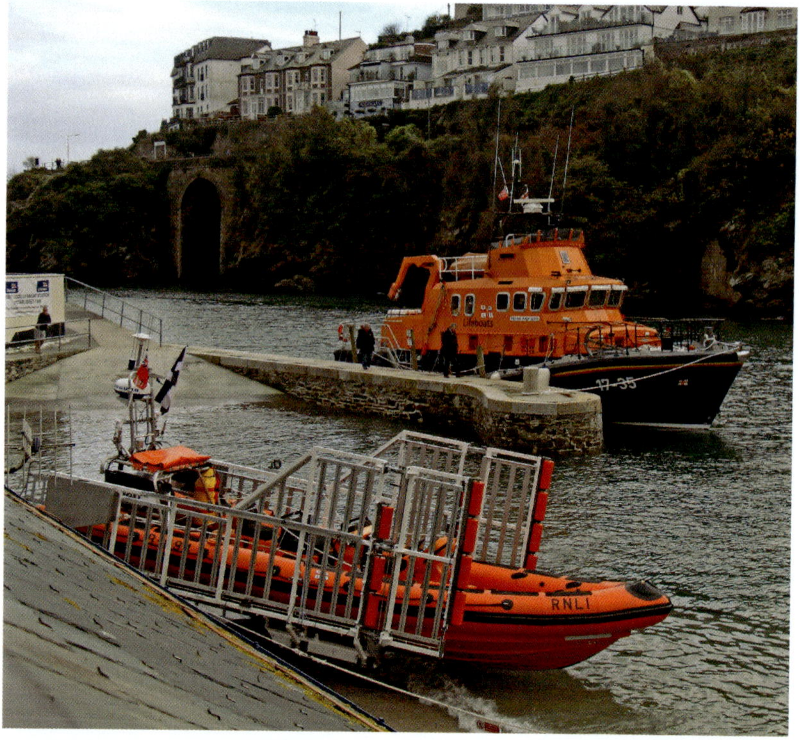

Fowey, Plymouth and Salcombe searching for a missing 18ft open fishing boat with two people aboard. The boat had gone out for an evening fishing trip but not returned home. Plymouth all-weather lifeboat was launched at 3.45am to search for the vessel, which had broken down and was lost in fog off the Eddystone. At around 8am both Atlantic and D class ILBs from Looe put out and both Fowey lifeboats also launched, being joined an hour later by Salcombe all-weather lifeboat.

The search was hampered by thick mist reducing visibility to less than 100m. The people on board the casualty vessel only had a mobile telephone, but after an extensive search they were spotted six miles south-west of the Eddystone lighthouse. The casualties were taken aboard the Plymouth lifeboat, the boat was towed in, and the lifeboats returned to their stations.

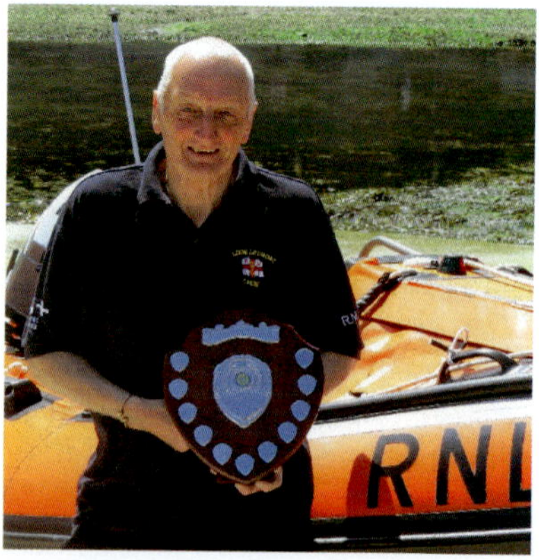

▶ In June 2018 LOM David Haines received an award for his voluntary work in Looe from the Rotary Club of Looe Valley. The award recognised his tireless work for the lifeboat station. David first volunteered for Looe RNLI when the station reopened in June 1992 and has been involved ever since. (Ian Foster)

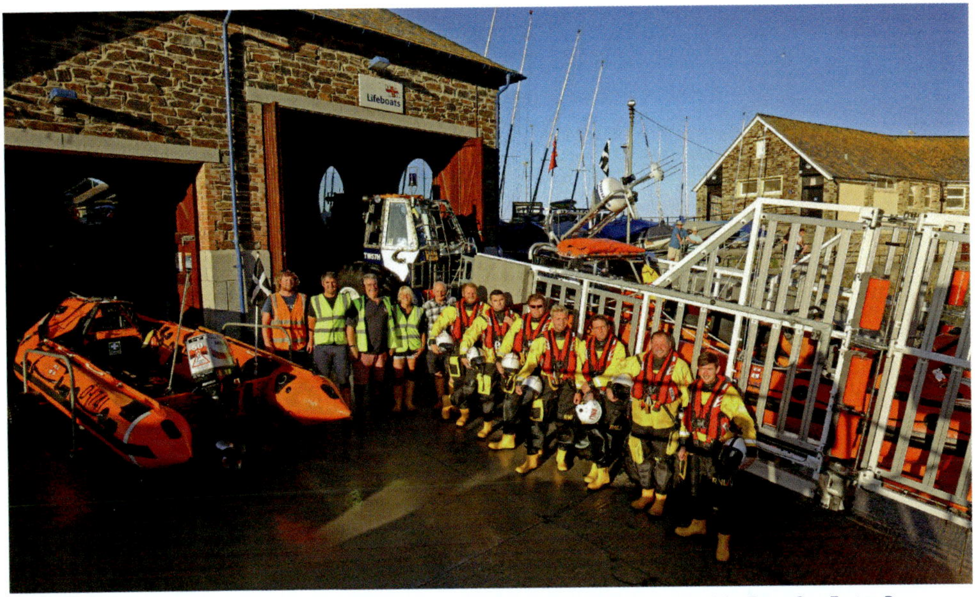

▲ Lifeboat crew and station personnel, June 2018, left to right: Jack Spree, David Jackman, John Pope, Sue Foster, Dave Haines (LOM), Nathaniel Rothwell, Dan King, Alastair Pearn, Goron Jones, Brian Bowdler, Clive Palfrey and Rob Deakin. This was one of Dan King's last training evenings, as he moved to the USA shortly afterwards. (Nicholas Leach)

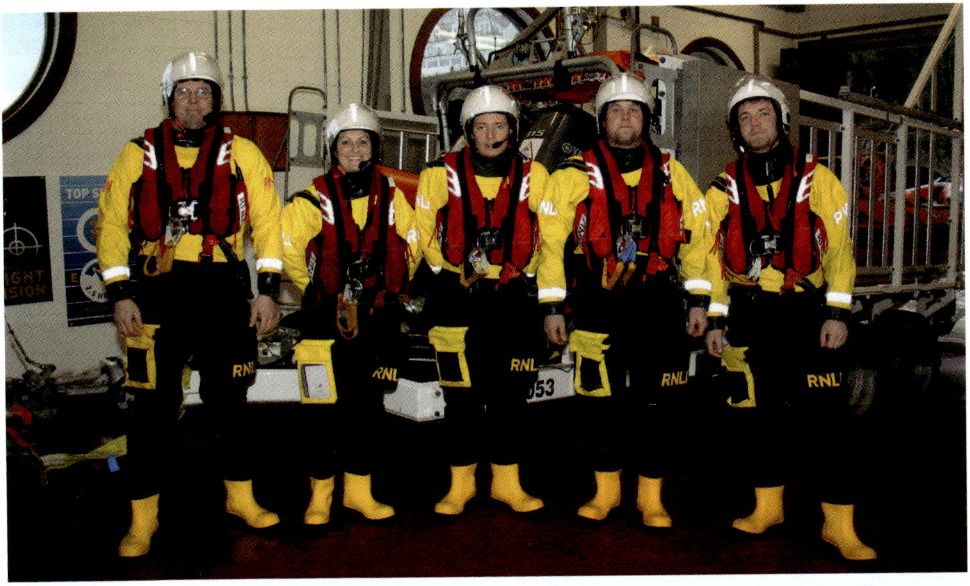

▲ Crew training and assessment at every RNLI lifeboat station is a continual process, and Looe is no exception with new crew being trained to the RNLI's high standards. On 6 March 2019, following several months of detailed training, RNLI Assessor Trainer Gary Stanbury visited Looe to formally assess five volunteer crew members, all of whom were formally passed out as substantive crew. The five crew were, left to right, Alastair Pearn, Victoria Thomas, Tom Peat, Jack Spree and Goron Jones. They were assessed on anchoring, search patterns, towing and several other aspects of boat handling. (Ian Foster)

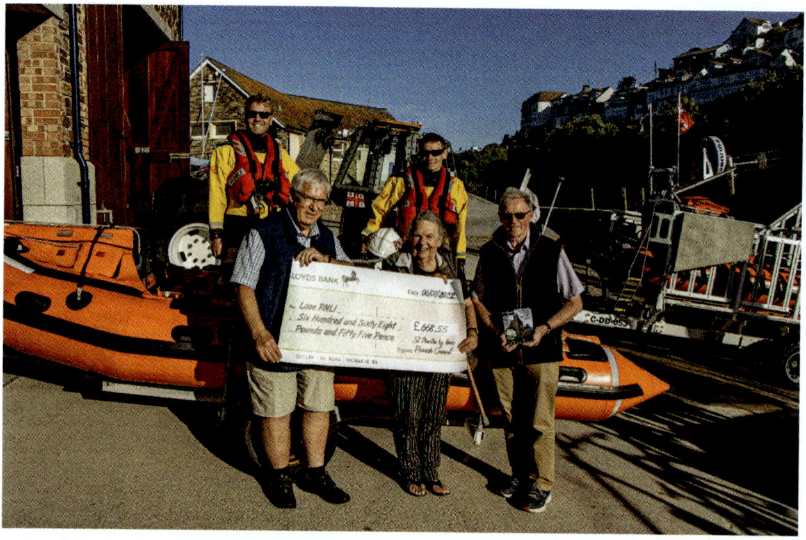

▶ Many people and organisation raise money for Looe lifeboat. On 6 July 2022 local historian Jenny Wallis, with Charles Hyde and Robert Henly, the clerk and chair of the parish council, visited the station to formally present a cheque For £668.55, the proceeds of the sale of Tithe maps sold through shop in the town. (Ian Foster)

Towards the end of the summer of 2016, on 7 September 2016, a new Atlantic 85, *Sheila & Dennis Tongue II* (B-894), was placed on station following a period of intensive crew training. She was one of four Atlantic 85 lifeboats funded by and named after Sheila and Dennis Tongue, who were both born in Birmingham, Dennis in 1929 and Sheila in 1927. Dennis became a product designer and later a senior manager at the company Valor. Sheila, despite serious illness as a young adult, enjoyed a career as a secretary and later obtained a degree in English from the Open University.

They were married in 1970 and upon Dennis' retirement moved to Devon to be by the coast. They began to appreciate the work of the RNLI, and how lifeboat stations are an integral part of a coastal town. They had no children and the decision to leave a substantial legacy to the RNLI was partly as a 'thank you' for the happy days they had spent in Exmouth and also in recognition of the work of the RNLI volunteers.

The new Atlantic 85 was formally named and dedicated at a ceremony on 12 November 2016 at the lifeboat station. The ceremony was overseen by John Tretheway, President of the station, and the

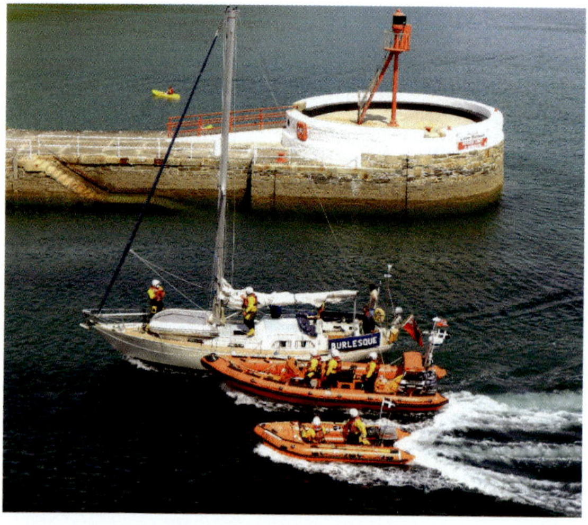

▼ Looe's lifeboats bringing in a yacht on 14 July 2020 after it had steering problems and was drifting in a strong offshore wind a mile and a half from Looe. (Ian Foster)

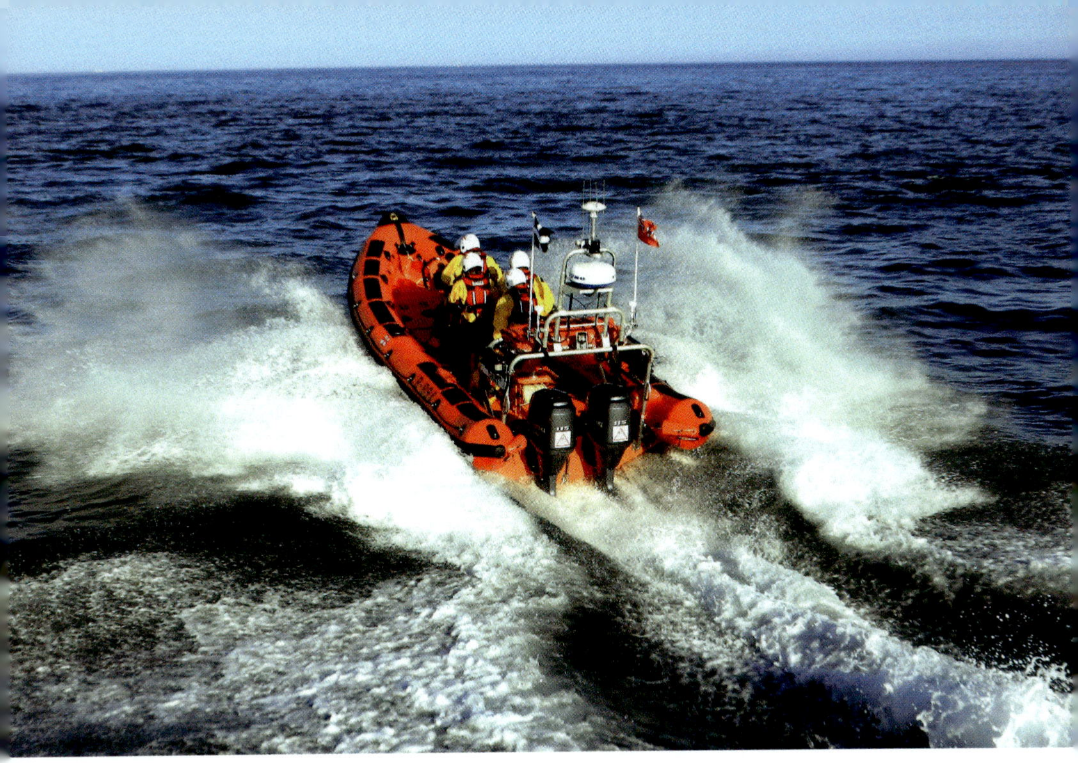

lifeboat was formally handed over by Raymond Tongue, representative of the donors. Following a service of dedication led by the Rev Philip Sharp and the Rev Andrew Hill, LOM David Haines invited Mr Tongue to name the lifeboat.

Since then, the Atlantic 85 and D class inflatable continue to undertake a variety of rescues. The challenges of rescue work were made more difficult in March 2020 when the first of several lockdowns came into force in order to combat the spread of the Covid-19 virus, but the lifeboats remained ready as before, and on 9 June 2020 both were launched after three persons got cut off by the tide between Looe and Portwrinkle. A search was started, and the crew on *Sheila and Dennis Tongue II*, shortly after arriving at Portwrinkle, spotted the casualties in a small cove. They were taken on board the lifeboat and returned safely to Looe.

A summer free of restrictions

▲ Atlantic 85 Sheila & Dennis Tongue II powers her way out of harbour. (Nicholas Leach)

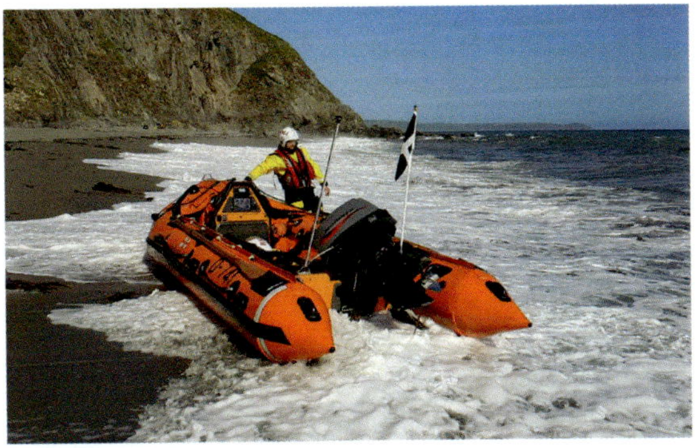

▲ The inshore lifeboat Ollie Naismith on the beach at Portwrinkle on 22 June 2020, with volunteer crew Toby Bray standing by. The ILB had been launched to help a female who had injured her leg after falling from a kayak. The lifeboat crew administered casualty care and took the female to a waiting ambulance at Portwrinkle harbour. (RNLI/Dan Margetts)

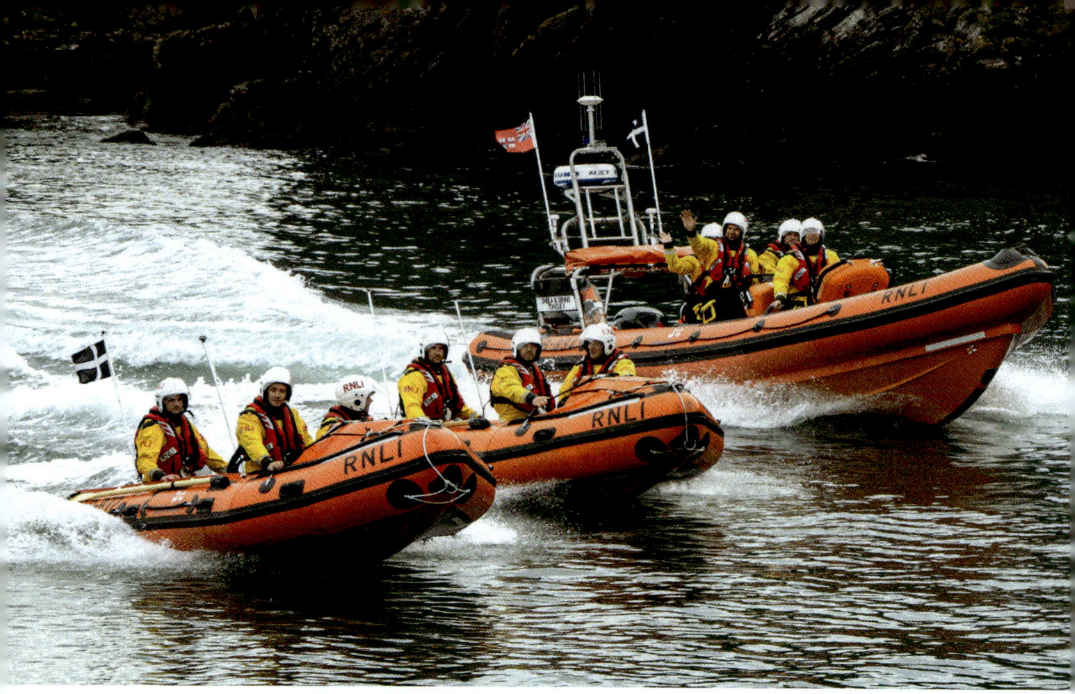

▲ Atlantic 85 Sheila & Dennis Tongue II (B-894) with Ollie Naismith (D-741) and Ollie Naismith II (D-872), 19 November 2022. Between December 2010 and November 2022 D-741 launched 236 times, assisted 165 people, and saved eight lives (Ian Foster)

in 2022 saw the beaches of Looe becoming busier and demands on the lifeboat volunteers were high. Among several rescues, on 12 August 2022 *Sheila and Dennis Tongue II* was launched to help three paddleboarders at the Longstone, east of Downderry, one of whom had sustained a shoulder injury. With no method of calling for help, one of the group paddled out to a local fishing boat, whose skipper contacted Falmouth coastguard and at 7.54am the Atlantic 85 was under way, finding the casualties in a small cove. All three were taken on board and returned to their vehicle, which was at Seaton beach, with the injured man making his own way to hospital.

Good teamwork between the rescue services was demonstrated on 14 October 2020 after *Ollie Naismith* went to help two persons cut off by the tide between Plaidy and Millendreath. Arriving on scene, the lifeboat crew located the casualties sitting on a cliff, just above breaking waves. Two attempts to extract them by veering the ILB down towards the cliff face were unsuccessful, due to the rocks and a four foot swell caused by the incoming tide. So Looe Coastguard Rescue team, who were on scene, lifted the casualties using ropes from the cliff top with the ILB standing by.

In March 2021 the RNLI announced an appeal to raise £78,000 to fund another new D class inflatable for the station. The appeal was launched during the pandemic so many traditional fundraising activities were on hold until restrictions had been relaxed, but nevertheless the community

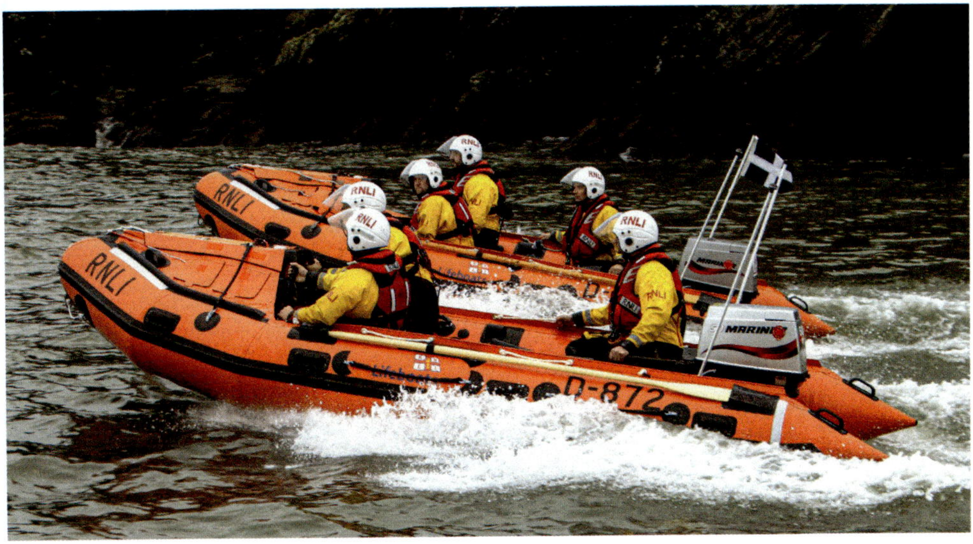

▲ The two Ollie Naismith ILBs together on 19 November 2022: the new boat D-872 on the inside, with D-741 behind. (Ian Foster)

responded magnificently and a range of activities were organised.

The outcome of the fundraising efforts was the new inshore lifeboat *Ollie Naismith II* (D-872), which was delivered to the station in November 2022, and officially placed on service at 12 noon on 19 November 2022. On the day, the new ILB and her predecessor, *Ollie Naismith* (D-741), were paraded together outside the lifeboat station, enabling the Naismith family to say farewell to the original boat while also welcoming the new ILB.

It was a unique opportunity for everyone to see both *Ollie Naismith* lifeboats together on the slipway and afloat on Looe river and Looe bay. In autumnal sunshine, Atlantic 85 *Sheila*

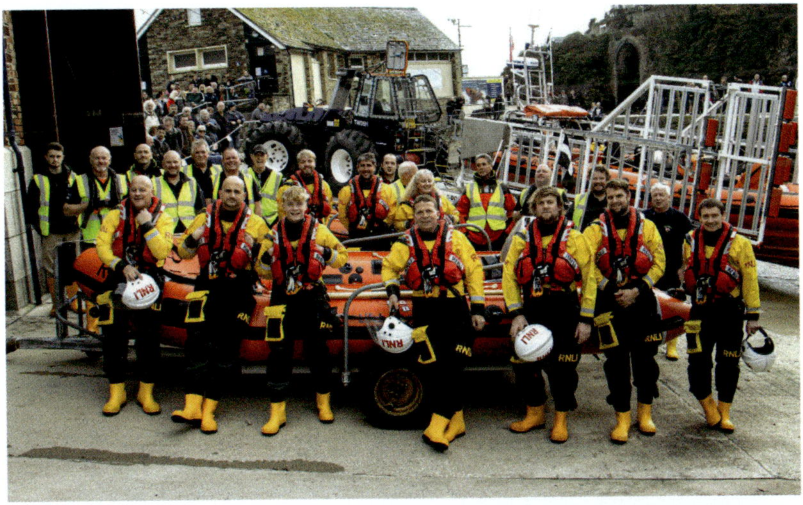

◀ Back, left to right: Jonty Wearing, Simon Rawe, John Goodsman, David Mitchell, David Robinson, Clive Palfrey, Nick Pope, Goron Jones, David Jackman, Eric Candy, David Haines, Victoria Thomas, Paul Barley, Del Palfrey, James Chudleigh, Ian Foster; front, left to right: Richard Porter, Toby Bray, Will Jaycock, Matt Jaycock, Jack Spree Richard Jones, Tom Peat. (Carol Foster)

and Dennis Tongue II was also launched to escort the two D class ILBs. Watching the lifeboats pass Ollie's memorial bench on the Banjo Pier, his father, John Naismith, commented:

'It was very emotional to see both lifeboats that have been named in memory of Ollie and today has been a day of great pride. I would like to thank everyone that had a part in this success, the achievement being even greater given the restrictions that Covid had on any activities when the Looe Lifeboat Appeal was launched.'

Ollie's mum, Maxine Naismith, his sister Tori, grandparents and other members of his family watched from the lifeboat station, and Maxine added: 'I am immensely grateful and proud of everyone at Looe RNLI for all the effort they made to honour the service and farewell ceremony for the *Ollie Naismith* lifeboat. We also welcomed *Ollie Naismith II* into service on Ollie's birthday. The occasion was a wonderful way to celebrate the enormous generosity and support our community and visitors gave to Looe RNLI. For me, it keeps Ollie at home in Looe. I am so very proud of his legacy and all the wonderful volunteer lifeboat crews.'

After the lifeboats were recovered, refuelled, washed down and made ready, Tom Mansell, the RNLI's Regional Lifesaving Lead, declared *Ollie Naismith II* was officially on service.

With their latest new ILB, the dedicated Looe lifeboat volunteers remain busy, guarding the coastline of south Cornwall. In 2022 the lifeboats were launched thirty-five times and nineteen persons were assisted, adding to the many people aided and lives saved since the station was reopened in 1992.

▼ Ollie Naismith II (D-872), pictured on 19 November 2022, is the sixth D class inflatable to serve Looe. (Ian Foster)

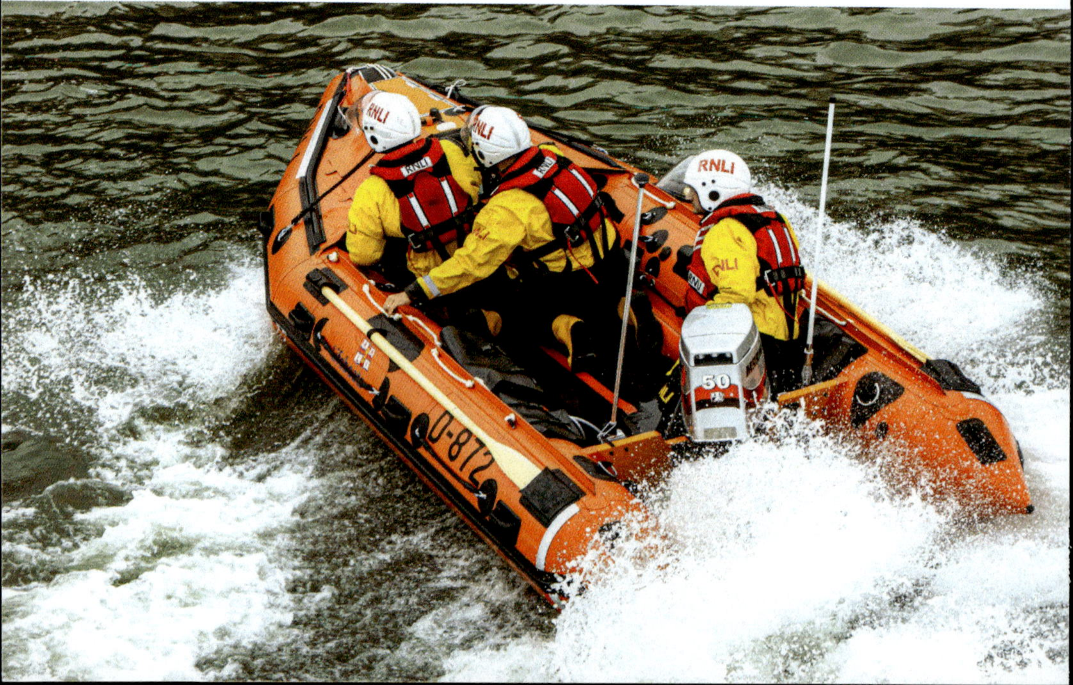

VOLUNTEER CREW AND STATION OFFICIALS 2023

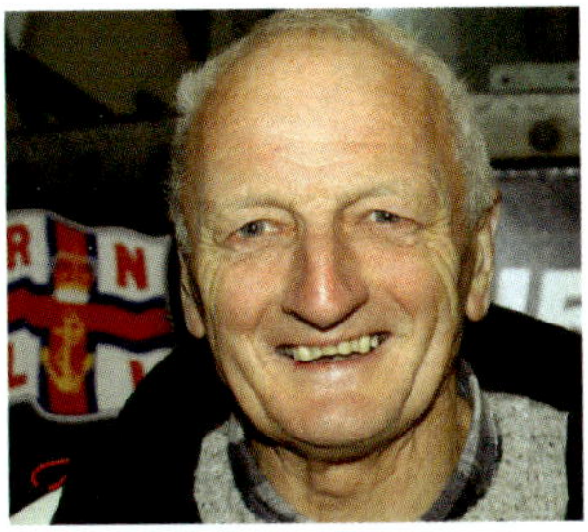

DAVID HAINES
Lifeboat Operations Manager

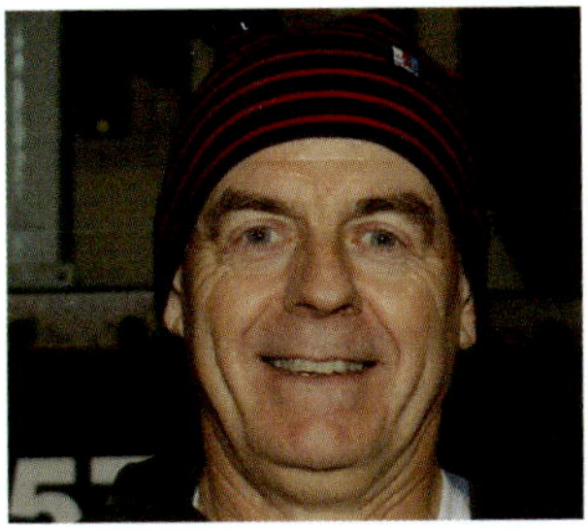

NICK POPE
Deputy Launching Authority

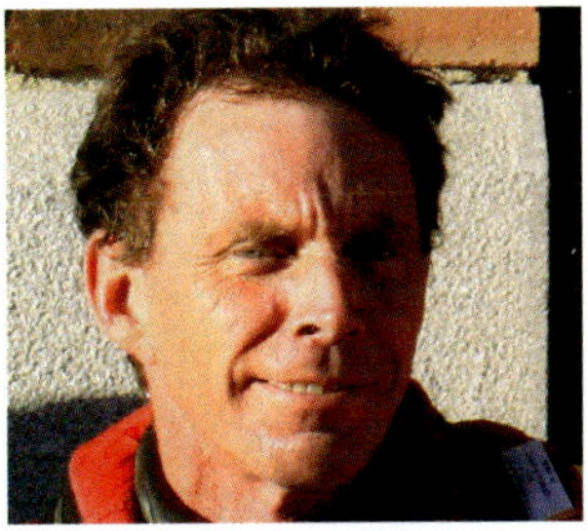

BRIAN BOWDLER
Deputy Launching Authority

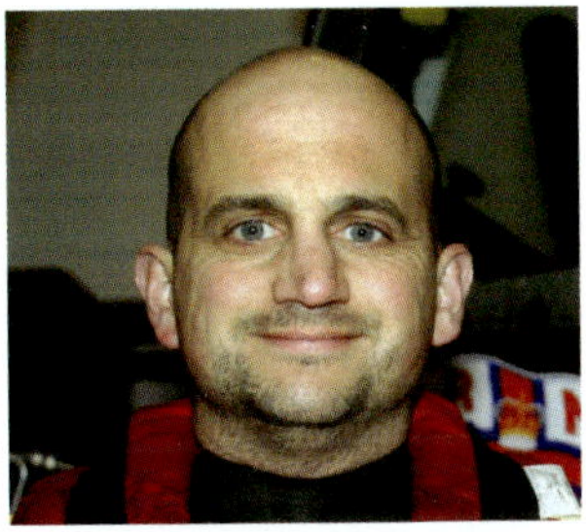

TOBY BRAY
ILB helm and station mechanic

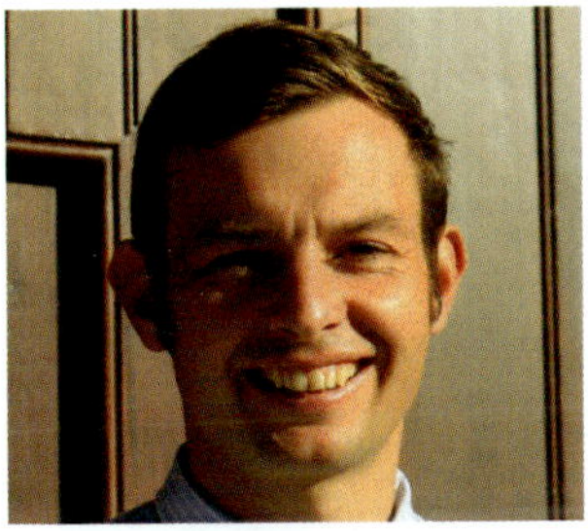

DAN MARGETTS
ILB helm and station mechanic

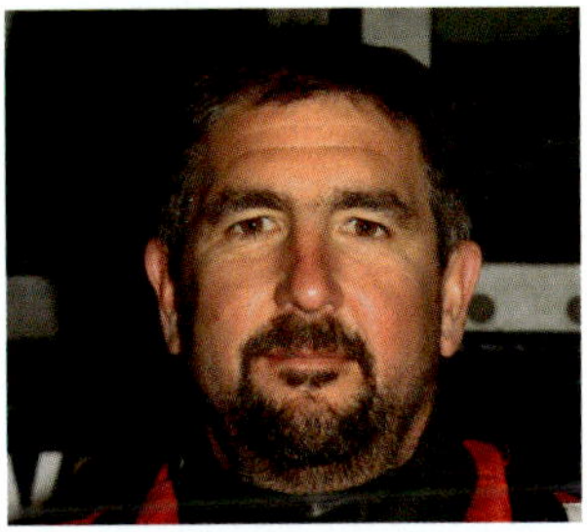

DAVID JACKMAN
ILB helm, training co-ordinator

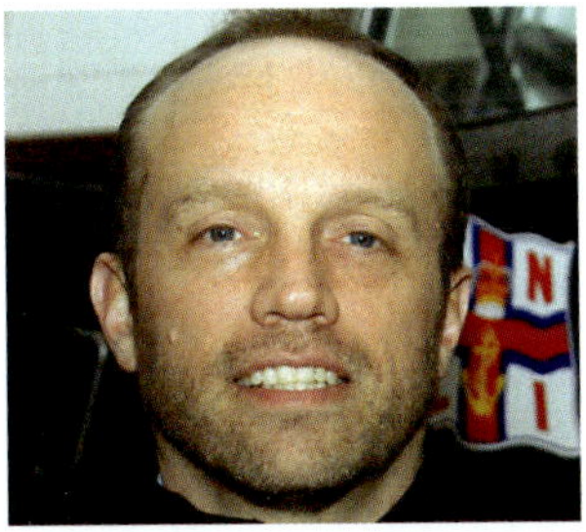

DALE STAFF
ILB crew, Lifeboat Medical Advisor

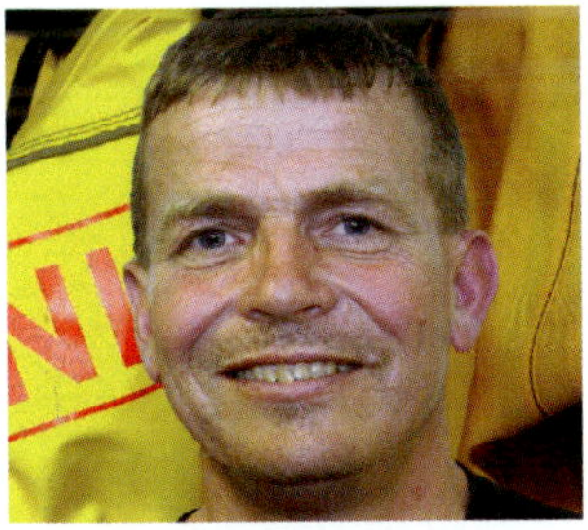

MATTHEW JAYCOCK
ILB helm and assessor/trainer

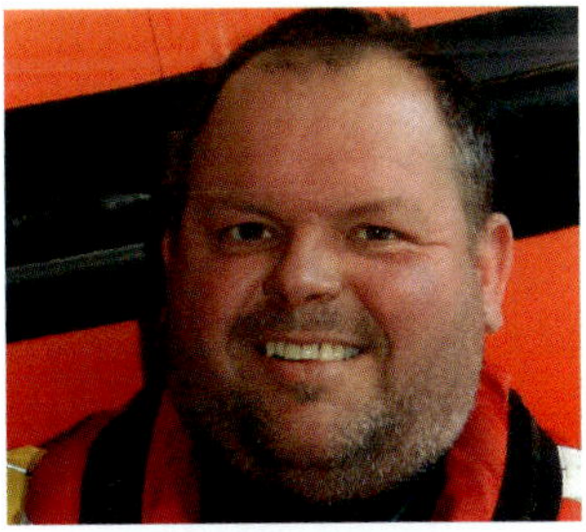

CLIVE PALFREY
ILB helm, training co-ordinator

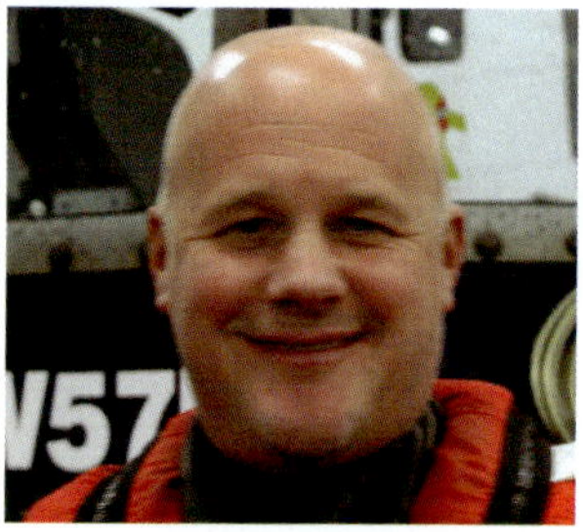

RICHARD PORTER
Trainee ILB helm and ILB crew

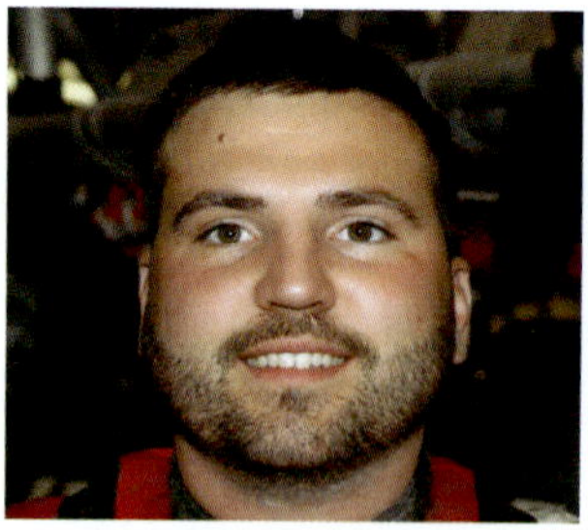

AARON RIX
Trainee ILB Helm and ILB crew

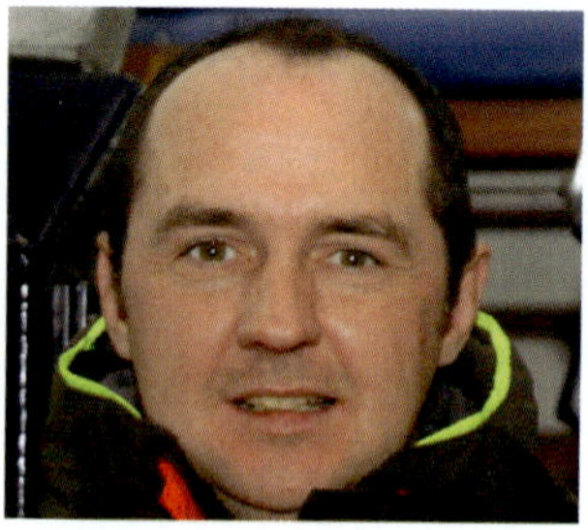

ERIC CANDY
Tractor driver, training co-ordinator

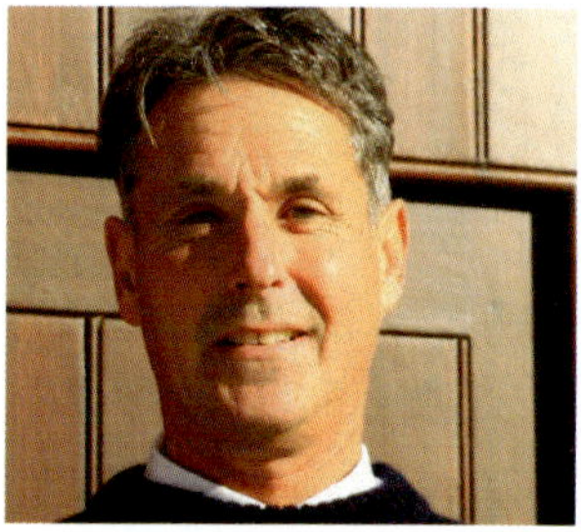

PAUL BARLEY
Tractor driver and shore crew

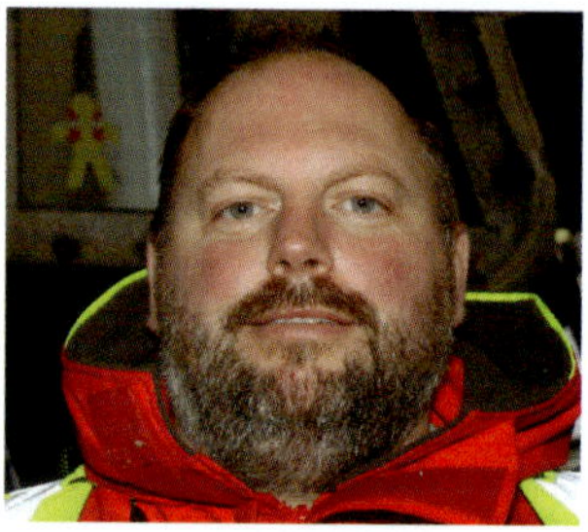

DEL PALFREY
Tractor driver and shore crew

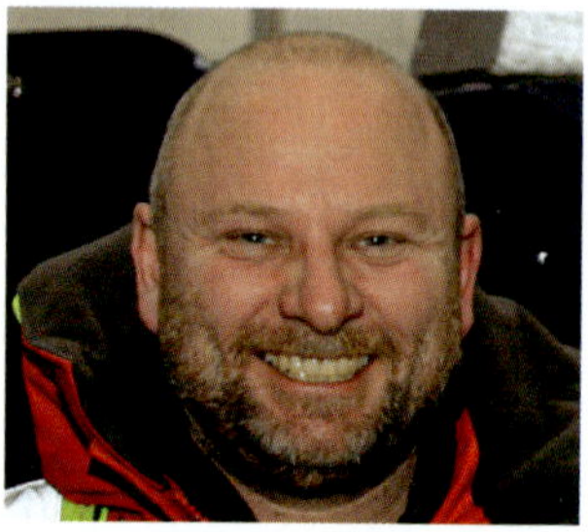

DAVID MITCHELL
Tractor driver and shore crew

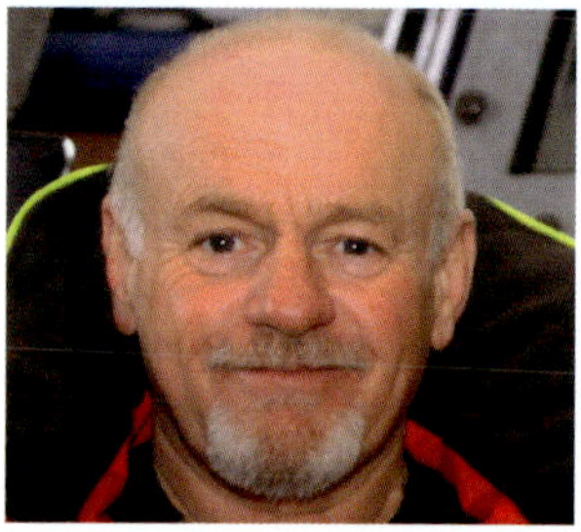

SIMON RAWE
Tractor driver and shore crew

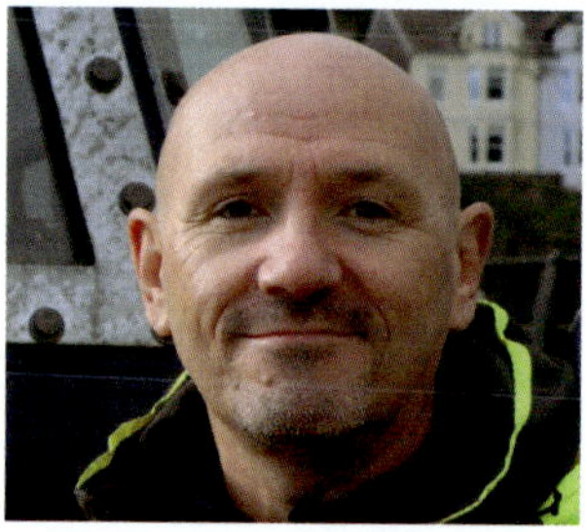

JOHN GOODSMAN
Tractor driver and shore crew

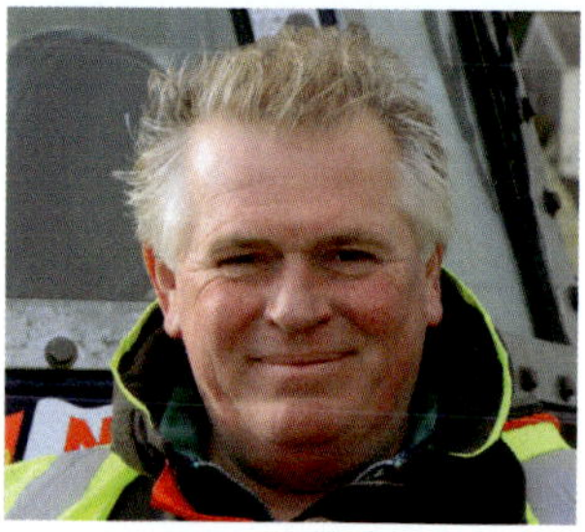

DAVID ROBINSON
Tractor driver and shore crew

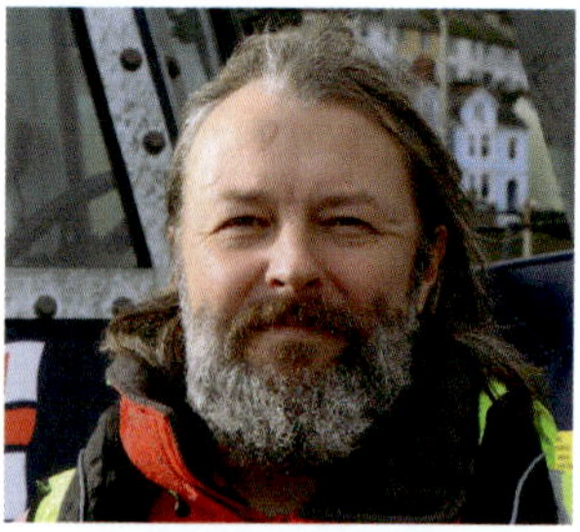

STUART HARESNAPE
Tractor driver and shore crew

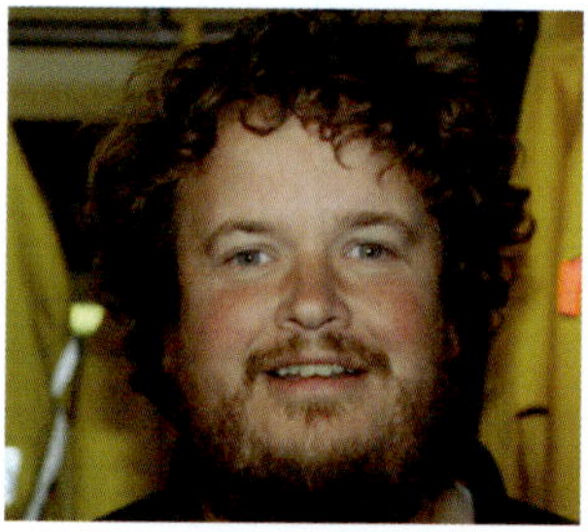

JAMES CHUDLEIGH
Shore crew

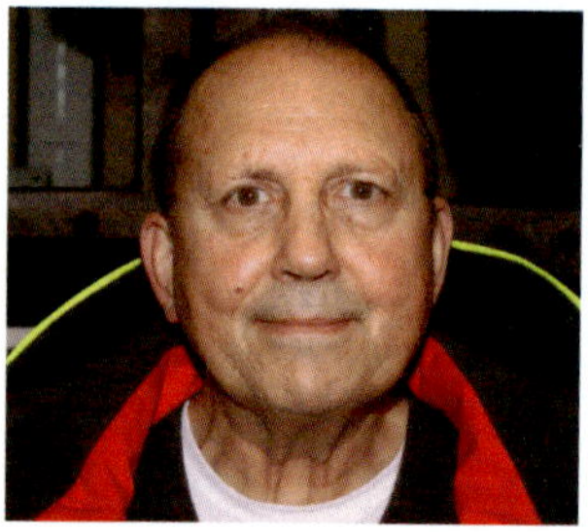

RICHARD RIX
Safety co-ordinator

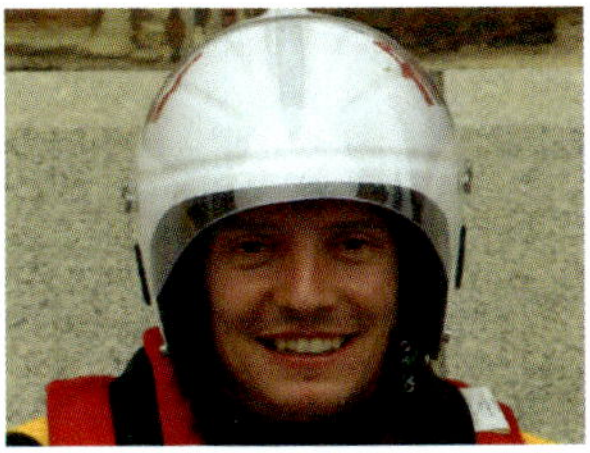

TOM PEAT
ILB crew

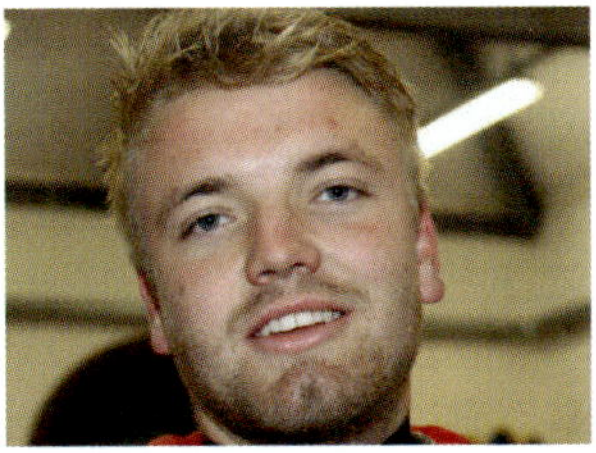

GORON JONES
ILB crew

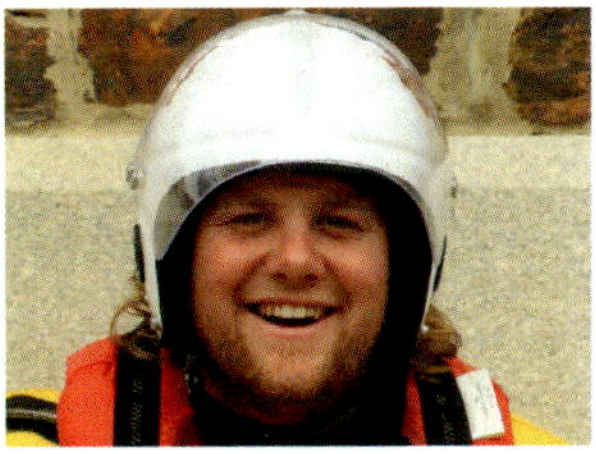

JACK SPREE
ILB crew

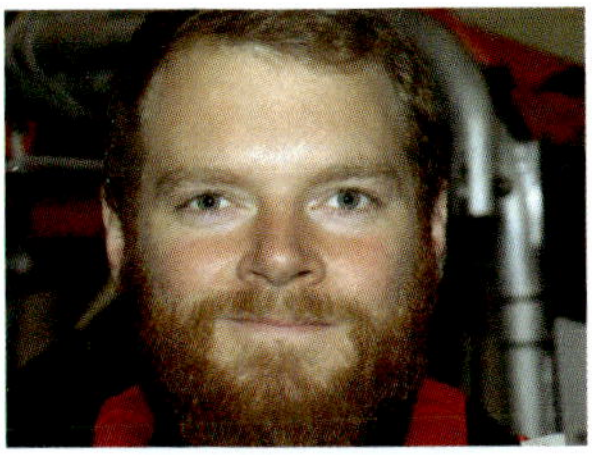

NATHANIEL ROTHWELL
ILB crew

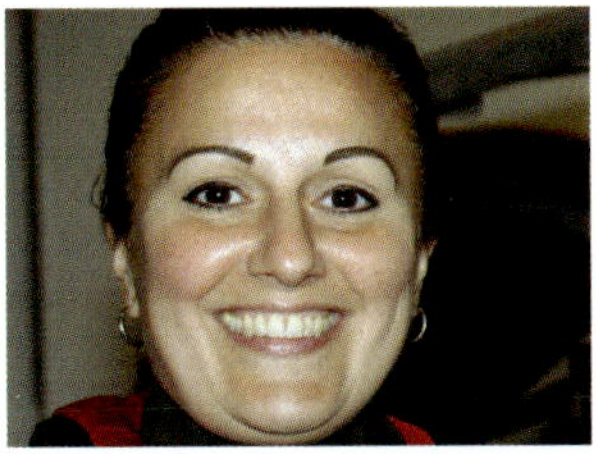

VICTORIA THOMAS
ILB crew

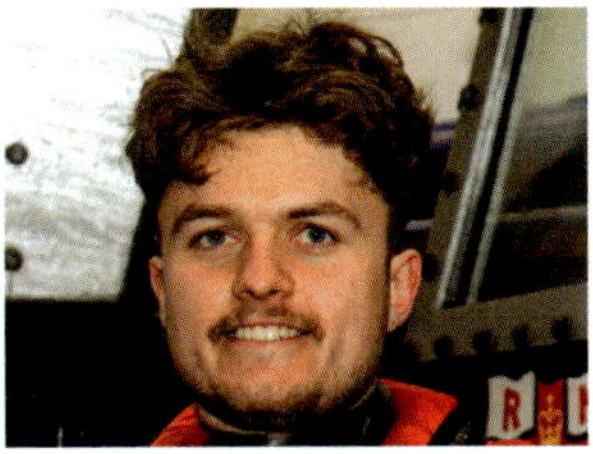

ALEX RICHARDSON
ILB crew

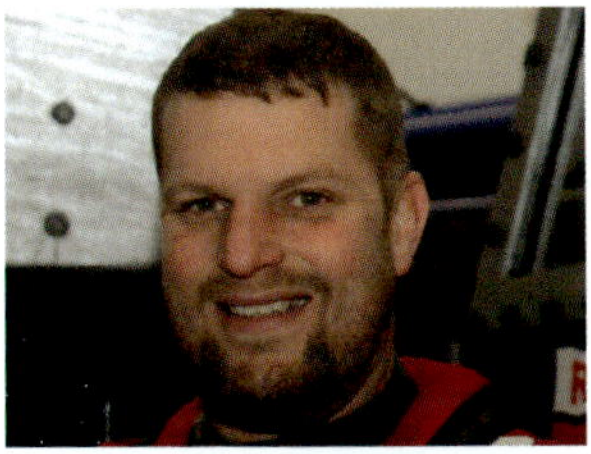

RICHARD JONES
ILB crew

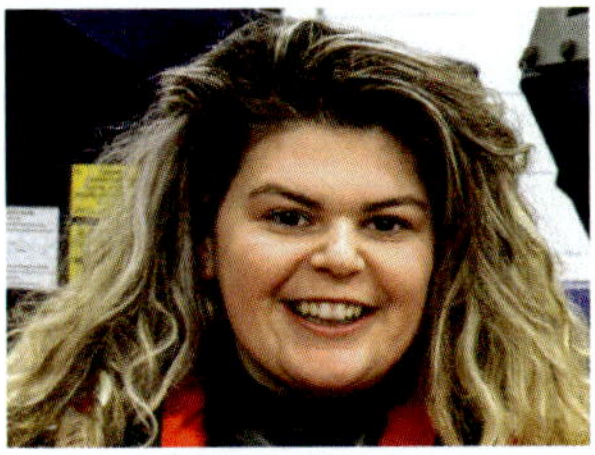

AMBER PALFREY
ILB crew

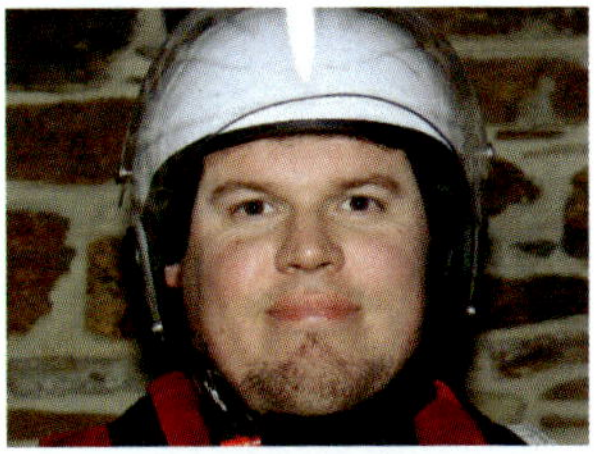

ALASTAIR PEARN
ILB crew

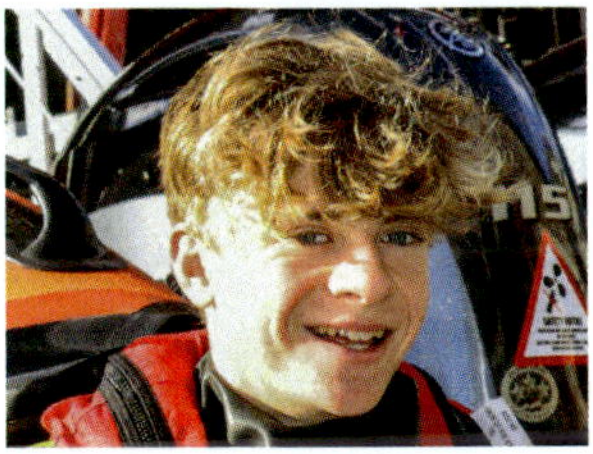

WILL JAYCOCK
ILB crew

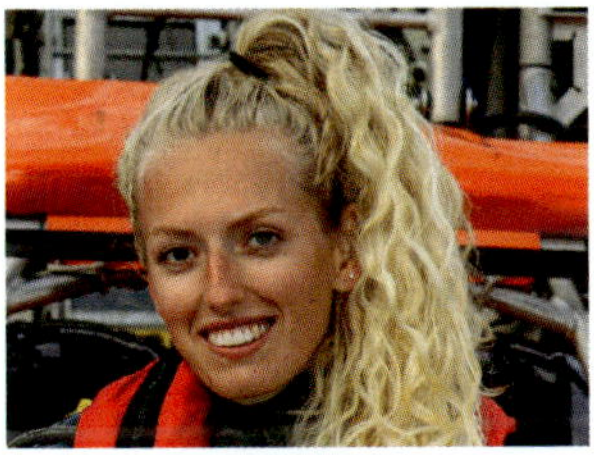

JENNIFER CREW
ILB crew

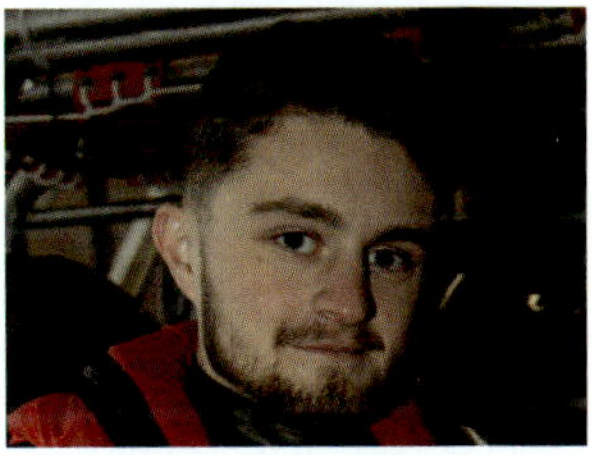

JONTY WEARING
Trainee ILB crew

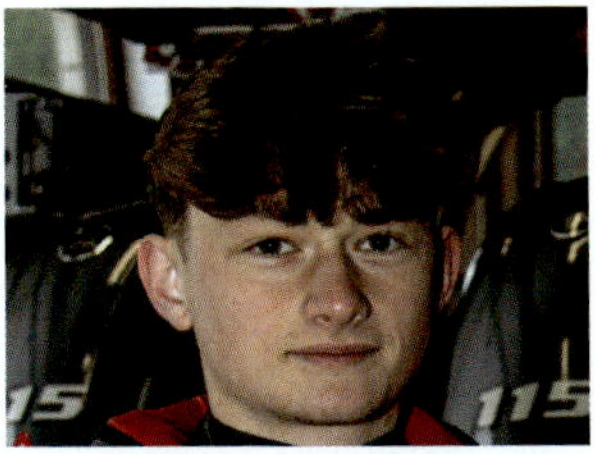

CHARLEY ANDERSON
Trainee ILB crew

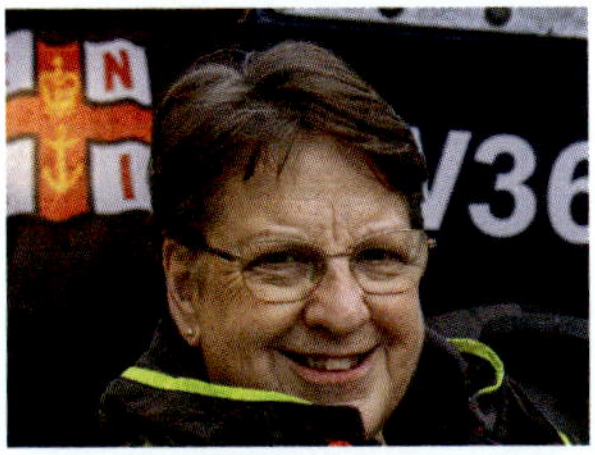

CAROL FOSTER
Lifeboat Visits Officer and shore crew

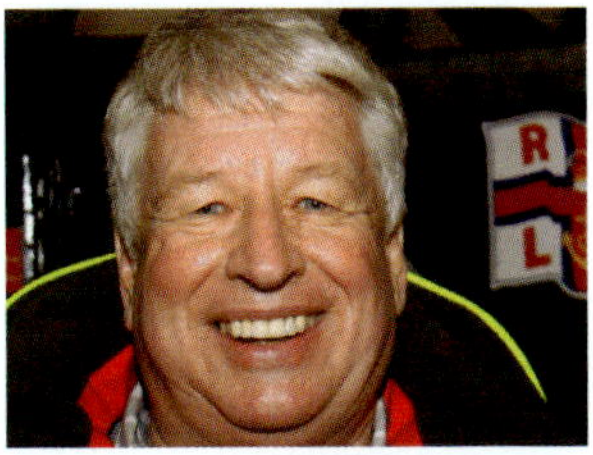

IAN FOSTER
Lifeboat Press Officer/shore crew

LAUNCHES AN

Year	Launches	Assisted
1992	11	13
1993	12	5
1994	14	5
1995	12	2
1996	16	13
1997	31	26
1998	21	10
1999	16	11
2000	31	31
2001	26	12
2002	28	34

Year	Launches	Assisted
2003	42	46
2004	26	15
2005	36	25
2006	32	35
2007	29	32
2008	34	28
2009	34	24
2010	49	33
2011	40	34
2012	44	39
2013	27	12

Year	Launches	Assisted
2014	63	30
2015	28	28
2016	36	32
2017	34	27
2018	33	16
2019	37	30
2020	40	49
2021	47	56
2022	35	19

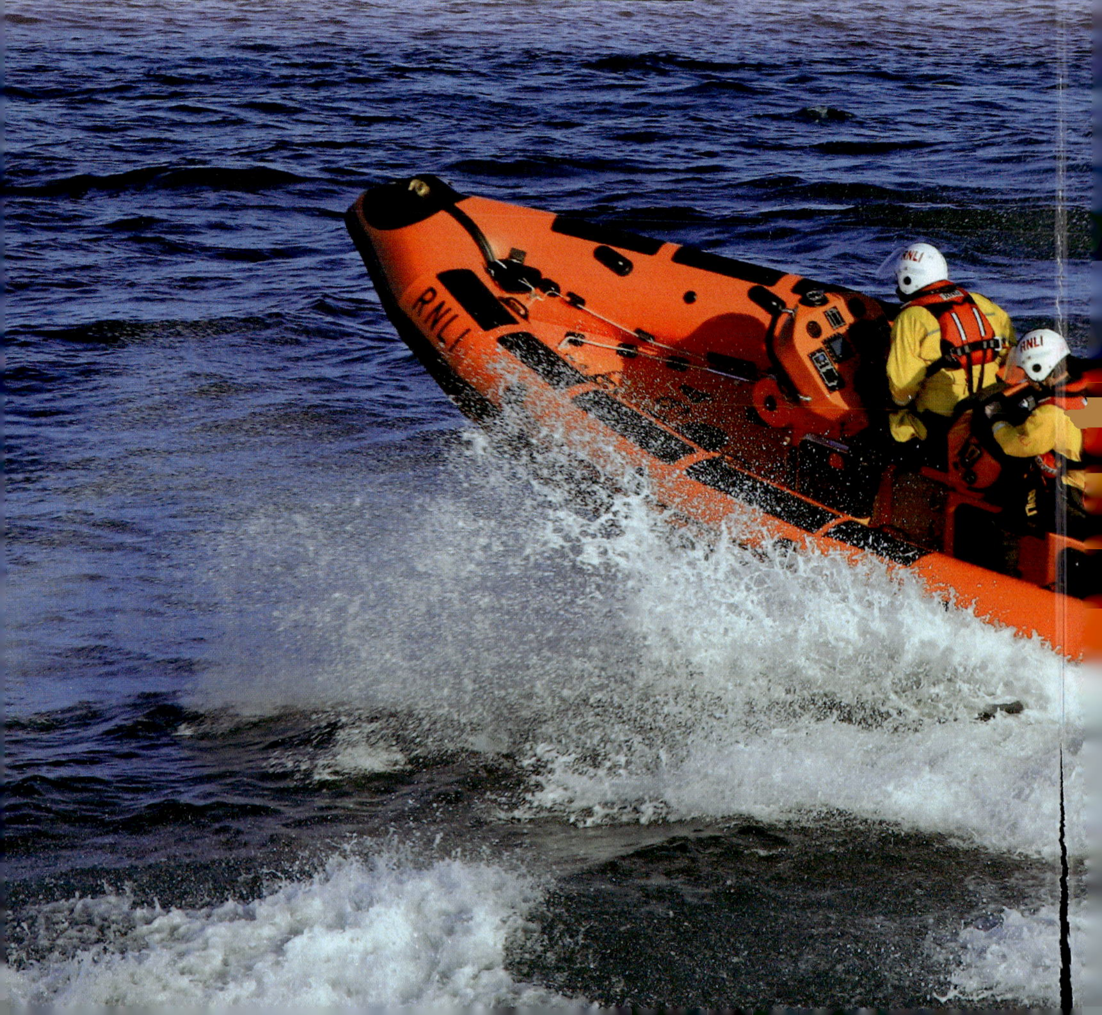

IVES SAVED

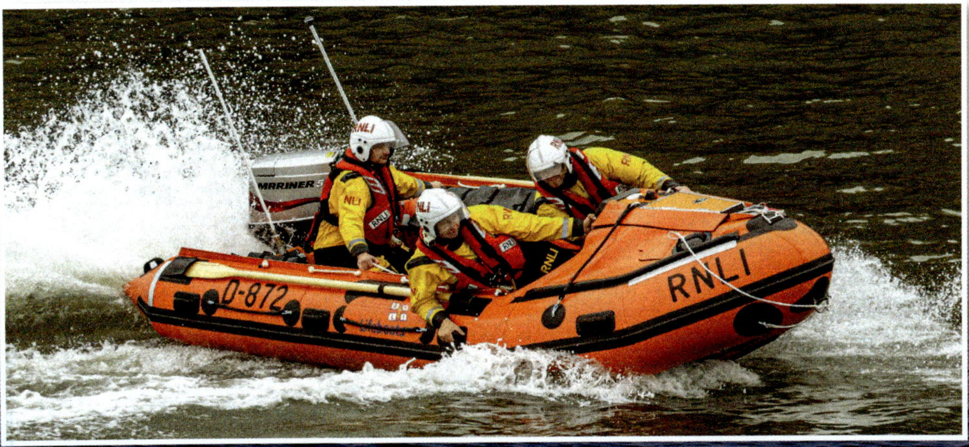

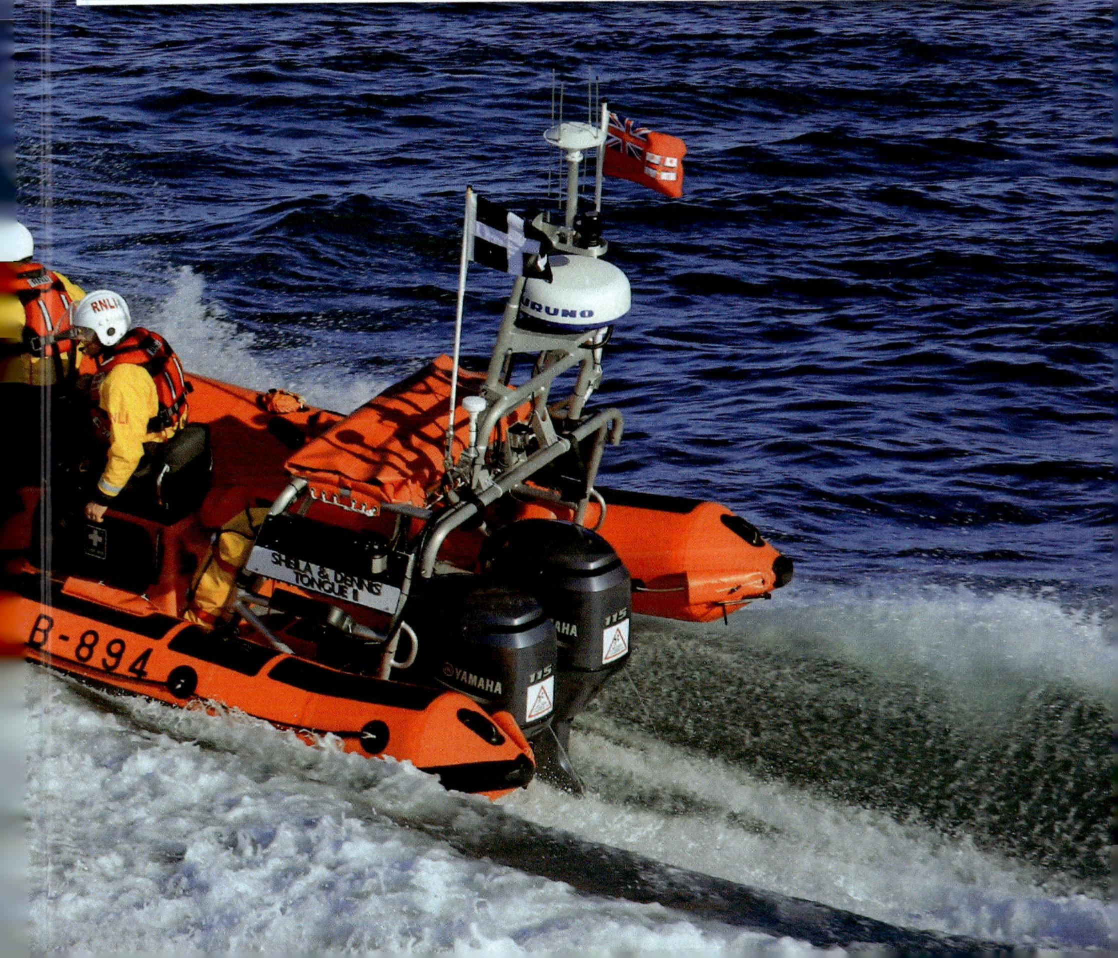

Pulling and Sailing Lifeboats

Years on station (launches/saved)	Dimensions Type	Cost ON	Year built Builder	Name Donor
12.1866 – 1882 (12/14)	32' x 7'6" Self-righter	£248 —	1866 Woolfe	*Oxfordshire* Gift of Sir John Pollard Willoughby, Bt
7.1882 – 5.1902 (7/23)	34' x 8' Self-righter	£329 45	1882 Woolfe	*Boy's Own No.1* Boy's Own Paper Lifeboat Fund
5.1902 – 31.7.1930 (12/37)	35' x 8'6" Self-righter	£835.17.0 489	1902 Thames IW	*Ryder* Legacy of William Ryder, Brixton

Inshore lifeboats

Years on station (launches/saved)	ON	Name (if any) Donor	Type
1991–94	D-355	— —	Avon EA16
1994	D-396	*Starting Point* Frizzell Insurance and Blakesley village	Avon EA16
1994–3.2002	D-461	*Spirit of the RAOC* Fund raising by the Royal Logistic Corps	Avon EA16
5.3.2002–11.2010	D-574	*Regina Mary* Gift of Laurence Allen	Avon EA16
15.11.2010–11.2022	D-741	*Ollie Naismith* Local appeal in memory of Ollie Naismith	IB1
20.11.2022–	D-872	*Ollie Naismith II* Local appeal in memory of Ollie Naismith	IB1
2.10.2003–9.2016	B-793	*Alan and Margaret* Gift of Miss Elizabeth Beaton	Atlantic 75
7.9.2016–	B-894	*Sheila & Dennis Tongue II* Legacy of Mr and Mrs Dennis Tongue, Birmingham	Atlantic 85

Personnel Record

Honorary Secretaries

Robert Thomas	1866-1894
Samuel Brock, Ch Off CG	1894-1898
Thomas Parson	1898-1900
Captain J.W. Hughes	1900-1905
Richard Harbord	1905-1908
John F. Chields	1908-1911
Captain John R. Barber	1911-1922
Colonel W.V. Moul	1922-1925
W.F. Phillips	1925-1930
- - - - - - - - - - - - - - - - - - - -	
Phillip Smallridge	5.1994-1996
Jonathan Brice	1996-12.2003
David Haines	12.2003-

Coxswains

William Alford	1866-3.1888
Albert Fisk	3.1888-1898
Edward Toms	1898-1919
William Thomas Toms	1919-1930

Second Coxswains

James Toms	1866-3.1888
Edward Toms	1888-1898
Percy Pearn	1898-1930 (?)